DR CHIARA HUNT AND MARINA FOGLE

The Bump Class

An Expert Guide to Pregnancy, Birth and Beyond

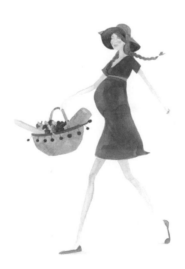

Contents

The
Bump Class

To our children, Ludo, Otto, Iona, Ivy and Willem, thank you for teaching us more about life, love, strength and resilience than we ever thought possible.

1 3 5 7 9 10 8 6 4 2

Vermilion, an imprint of Ebury Publishing,
20 Vauxhall Bridge Road,
London SW1V 2SA

Vermilion is part of the Penguin Random House group of companies whose addresses can be found at global.penguinrandomhouse.com

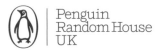

Penguin
Random House
UK

Text © Marina Fogle and Chiara Hunt 2016
Illustrations © Leonora Williams-Wynne 2016
Photograph on page 255 © Helene Sandberg 2015

Marina Fogle and Chiara Hunt have asserted their right to be identified as the authors of this Work in accordance with the Copyright, Designs and Patents Act 1988

First published by Vermilion in 2016

www.eburypublishing.co.uk

A CIP catalogue record for this book is available from the British Library

ISBN 9780091959739

Colour origination by Rhapsody Ltd London
Printed and bound in China by Toppan Leefung

Penguin Random House is committed to a sustainable future for our business, our readers and our planet. This book is made from Forest Stewardship Council® certified paper.

The information in this book has been compiled by way of general guidance in relation to the specific subjects addressed, but is not a substitute and not to be relied on for medical, healthcare, pharmaceutical or other professional advice on specific circumstances and in specific locations. So far as the authors are aware the information given is correct and up to date as at: August 2015. Practice, laws and regulations all change, and the reader should obtain up to date professional advice on any such issues. The authors and publishers disclaim, as far as the law allows, any liability arising directly or indirectly from the use, or misuse, of the information contained in this book.

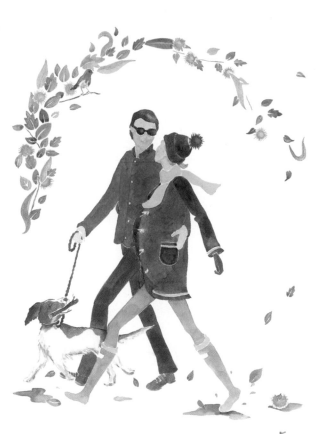

You and Your Baby

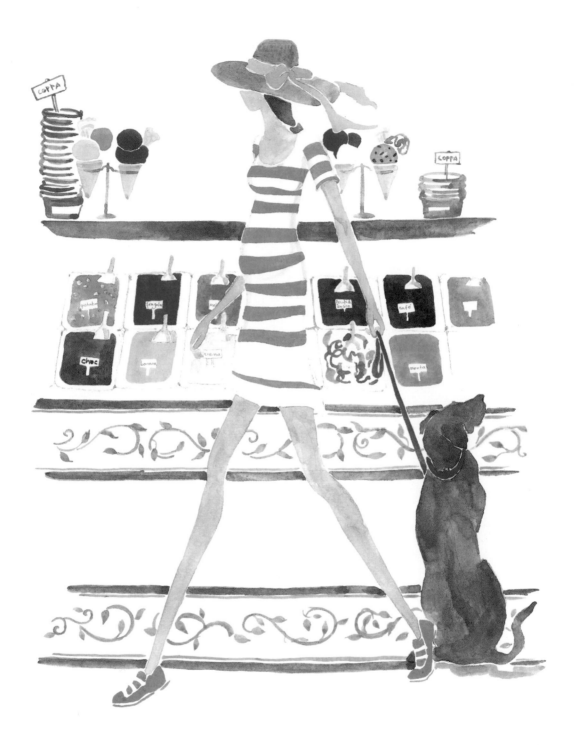

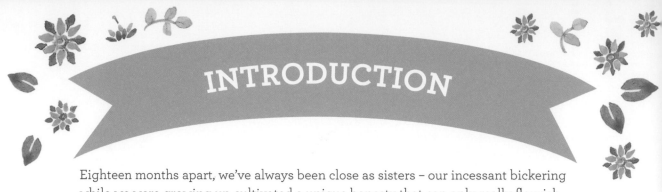

INTRODUCTION

Eighteen months apart, we've always been close as sisters – our incessant bickering while we were growing up cultivated a unique honesty that can only really flourish when you have absolutely no hesitation to tell the other how annoying they are being. But the whole experience of having children, supporting each other through the anguish of loss, the joy of new life and the pain of deadly fatigue brought us closer still and now sees us not only run a business, but spend virtually every weekend together, to the extent that our four children regard each other as siblings rather than cousins.

What we've realised supporting each other, good friends and the girls on The Bump Class – the ante- and postnatal class that we set up and now run together – is that pregnancy and birth is always different. Some women sail through their pregnancies, glowing and relishing every moment and others feel rotten, scared, out of control or just debilitated by sickness. One group are not going to fare better than the other, it's just the way it is and it applies to birth too. For the majority of women, birth is straightforward, natural and our bodies do what they were built for flawlessly. But for others it is more of a challenge and for a variety of reasons, they might need some help. Again, the first group have not done better than the second group; to give birth, however it happens, is a remarkable achievement and as long as both mothers and babies are safe there is no time for any mother to feel guilty or ashamed about how the birth itself went.

There seems to be an alarming trend for doctors to be regarded as the enemy when it comes to birth and this really could not be further from the truth. The decision to intervene by a doctor is not made because he wants to finish up and get to the pub or needs more practice with forceps. The decision is based on the wellbeing of mother and baby, because birth is still a risky business. Worldwide childbirth is still one of the leading causes of death in adult women. In the UK this is not the case because we have hospitals, midwives and doctors who use their skills to ensure the vast majority of babies are delivered safely into their parents' arms.

Do doctors sometimes intervene too quickly? Yes – there are often cases where with hindsight intervention is subsequently deemed unnecessary. But doctors do not have the luxury of hindsight when they are making a split second decision. Surely it is best that we are cautious and risk averse, than cavalier with a higher number of negative outcomes.

But it can be a scary process – even if birth goes beautifully and there are no complications, it can be a frightening experience if you are not prepared for it. The

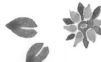

old adage, knowledge is power, is never more true than for women expecting their first babies. We believe that the best thing you can do in your pregnancy is to acquaint yourself with what is happening at each stage of your pregnancy, understand why the various tests, scans and checks are being performed, know about the physiology of labour and the terms used both when it is straightforward or slightly more complicated, and finally know about and understand what potential medical interventions may be necessary. If you are able to do all this then the moment your baby is born, whether in the birth pool or in the operating theatre, will be one of the most magical moments of your life.

When we first conceived The Bump Class the thing we were most adamant about was wanting to give honest, practical but above all professional advice. The spectrum of information is so wide we did not want to rely on simply one professional's expertise, but rather a variety of leaders in their field who could communicate, with charisma and an element of fun, the knowledge so essential for mothers to be. This book is no different and we have gleaned the expertise of trusted specialists – physiotherapists, midwives, obstetricians, anaesthetists, breastfeeding specialists and paediatricians. It is because we have included this spectrum of specialists that we feel that this book is unique.

With all the experiences that we are privileged enough to be a part of we realised very quickly that the words 'always' and 'never' with regards to what is normal should not be used. While there are guidelines to which the majority of women adhere, as humans we are much more complex than even science currently understands and when it comes to pregnancy and birth, there will always be exceptions to the rule. Throughout this book we have tried to explain what the normal is, but everything should be read with the understanding that there is always the exception.

As exciting as it is for a woman to learn that there is a little being inside her, with a heartbeat from very early on, we do not refer to a baby until 24 weeks' gestation. Clinically it is an embryo until 9 weeks, a fetus until 24 weeks and from then, when theoretically a baby can live outside the uterus, a baby. We know from both personal and professional experience how losses are common in the early days and then become less likely as the pregnancy progresses. But pregnancy is hard enough, so it's perhaps a good idea not to think of your baby as a little person until you are well into your pregnancy.

For the last year, we have worked late into the night, our children asleep in the same room, or grabbed precious moments when all four played harmoniously, writing this book, all the while cementing our knowledge through the myriad of emotions that comes with pregnancy and motherhood and through the experiences The Bump Class have shared with us. It has brought us closer still. In fact our children summed our relationship up pretty well one afternoon when we were all in the car together, our four chatterboxes debating what 'being married' was. We established that Grandma was married to Grandpa and Opi to Omi. 'So who is Auntie Marina married to?' Chiara asked. For a moment there was silence as each of them pondered the question. 'Auntie Chiara?' asked Iona.

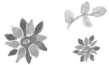

1 The 40 weeks of *pregnancy timeline*

Pregnancy is dated over 40 weeks and consists of three trimesters – essentially three lots of roughly three months. This may seem rather confusing though, as you're not actually pregnant for 40 weeks …

embryo size

WEEKS

Your pregnancy is dated from the first day of your last period …

1

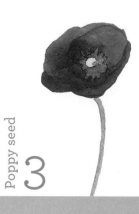

Poppy seed

3

The beginning of week 5 is when your next period would be due. This is usually when people first realise they're pregnant and when you can do a pregnancy test.

5

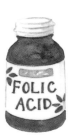

2

… although conception will have only occurred sometime between weeks 2 and 3. As sperm can live up to seven days, and an egg 24 hours, actual conception might have occurred a few days after intercourse.

Sesame seed

4

Did you know (with very rare exceptions) there is no such thing as a false positive, so if the test says you're pregnant, you almost definitely are. However, if the result is negative, you may still be preganant and may even test positive on the next test.

Chocolate chip

6

The first trimester

This trimester is when most of your baby's development is happening so do be aware of what you're eating and drinking. For a lot of girls, the first trimester is the worst: you tend to feel awful and you're reluctant to tell anyone. Most people start to feel tired and sick from weeks 6 to 9. This is made worse by the fact that a lot of people want to keep their pregnancy a secret until they reach 12 weeks, so there's no sympathy either ...

At week 9 your embryo graduates to being a fetus.

Blueberry
7

Gummy Bear
8

Olive
9

Plum
10

Golfball
11

Lime
12

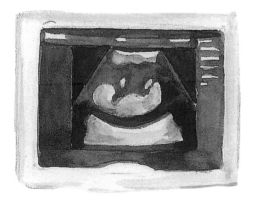

At week 12, you may be able to hear the fetus' heartbeat with a doppler.

Week 12 is when you have your first really important scan: the nuchal scan (see page 50).

The second trimester

This is generally when the pregnancy glow kicks in. Any morning sickness should ease by around week 15 and you'll notice your skin start to glow and your hair may start to thicken. Finally you can share your exciting news with friends and family. Enjoy this time – most people agree that this is when they enjoy their pregnancy the most.

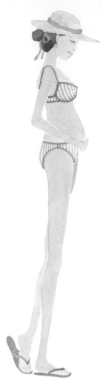

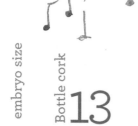

By week 15 an ultrasonographer should be able to determine the sex of your fetus.

WEEKS

embryo size

Bottle cork **13**

Onion **15**

Turnip **17**

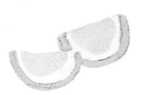

Lemon **14**

Avocado **16**

Bell pepper **18**

No visible bump yet? Don't worry, a lot of first time mothers don't look very pregnant until after 20 weeks.

Studies suggest that fetuses can start to hear at 16 weeks although the ears are not fully developed until 24 weeks.

Around week 18 most mothers start to feel little fluttery movements of their fetuses.

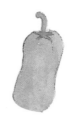

Your fetus has eyelashes and fingernails by week 19.

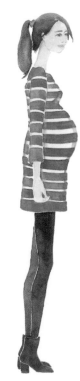

19

Carrot ## 21

Mango ## 23

25

Small banana ## 20

Week 20 is when the second really important scan is performed – the anomaly scan (see page 72). Here all your fetus' organs and structures will be looked at in detail to check they're present and correct.

Grapefruit ## 22

Corn on the cob ## 24

If your baby is born after 24 weeks she has a reasonable chance of survival.

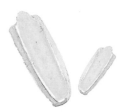

26

The third trimester

In the final trimester pregnancy becomes tiring, and as you near the end you may start to feel fed up. Sleep starts to become more difficult as it's harder to get comfortable and you'll notice some swelling in your legs and fingers. As your baby has less space to move, she starts putting pressure on your organs, which can be uncomfortable. But the good news is that it won't be long now until you meet your baby.

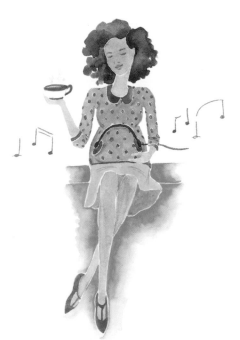

By week 29 your baby's bones, although soft, are fully developed.

By 27 weeks your baby can open her eyes.

embryo size

Cauliflower

27

Butternut squash

29

Large coconut

31

Pineapple

33

Romaine lettuce

35

WEEKS

Aubergine

28

Large cabbage

30

32

34

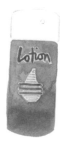

Lotion

From 37 weeks you're considered 'term', which means if your baby was born now she would not be premature.

Small watermelon

Most first babies are born at around 41 weeks.

37

39

41

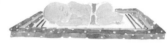

Leek

36

38

Small pumpkin

40

42

Most airlines will not let you fly after 36 weeks (or 32 weeks if you're carrying twins). You will need a letter from your doctor if you plan to fly after 28 weeks.

In the UK your due date is calculated at 40 weeks but actually less than 5 per cent of babies are born on their due date.

It's not considered safe to let a pregnancy go beyond 42 weeks, so by now your baby will have arrived!

2 Common *pregnancy myths*

'If your bump is low you're having a boy, and if it's high and wide it's a girl'

Neither of us found out the sex of our children before they were born and every time there was endless speculation about the sex. Our mother observed our bumps and only on one occasion predicted correctly. The reality is there is no evidence to show that the sex of the baby can be predicted from the shape of your bump, the beauty (or lack thereof) of the mother or the fetal heart rate.

One saying claims that bad morning sickness means you're having a boy. In fact, the opposite is more likely to be true. Research has shown that women carrying girls are more likely to have higher levels of hCG, the pregnancy hormone which causes nausea, so, if anything, being horribly sick means you're more likely to be carrying a girl.

Research suggests that the one other thing that might indicate the baby's sex is maternal instinct. Of all of the studies done into predicting gender, the mum's instinct is the one with the more convincing statistics. And don't forget: anyone's guess is 50 per cent likely to be correct!

'Before ultrasound could predict the sex of the baby, the story goes that an obstetrician would say that he always predicted the sex of the baby correctly. He'd tell the parents his prediction and then write down the opposite in their notes. If he had guessed correctly, the parents would return to him, impressed that he'd been correct. If he was wrong, he'd bring out his notes and say, "No, I told you it would be a boy. You see I wrote it down in your notes!"' CHIARA

'Listening to classical music in the uterus will mean my child will be clever'

During the 1980s a researcher suggested that playing classical music to your bump in the final stages of pregnancy boosted the intelligence of the child. Subsequent studies have not been so convincing, and for the time being there is little evidence to show that this would benefit your baby in any way. That's not to say that spending a bit of time relaxing and listening to classical music in your pregnancy is not going to benefit you or your baby. If it relaxes you, there's no doubt your baby will benefit. That said, if you prefer Coldplay, Desert Island Discs or hypnobirthing, they're probably just as beneficial.

'Pregnant women develop "baby brain"'

A lot of mothers (including us) feel that pregnancy made them more forgetful. Although studies have shown that mothers' brains do shrink towards the end of pregnancy, there is no evidence to show whether this has any effect on its performance. It may be that subtle changes in the brain are preparing mothers for the new challenges of motherhood. So while women may suffer in some areas, like remembering what has just been said to them, they may benefit in other areas, such as remembering information already stored in the brain. Studies have shown that heavily pregnant women seem to become less stressed, possibly as the result of increased levels of oestrogen. Regardless of why and how it happens, managing to stay calm is without doubt an invaluable skill for motherhood.

'Women with large feet have easy births'

For those of you who have spent years squeezing your feet into pretty little shoes, we're afraid there is no silver lining to having large feet when it comes to childbearing. A study was carried out that took women's height, weight and shoe size into account and there was no correlation between any of these and the length of labour. More likely to influence this is whether or not the baby is engaged when it all starts, which way the baby is facing, the size of your baby and the size and shape of your pelvis. The expression 'child-bearing hips' is unfair as it suggests that pear-shaped women might have easy births. In fact it's the size of your pelvic opening, rather than the width of your hips, that could determine how easy your labour is.

3 Finding out you *are pregnant*

Seeing that little '+' sign emerge on your pregnancy test is an emotional time for every woman, regardless if the pregnancy is unexpected or desperately wanted. Most people find out they're pregnant when they miss a period, making them approximately four weeks pregnant.

In order to date your pregnancy and work out your due date, you count 40 weeks from the first day of your last period. Bear in mind that if you have irregular periods your estimation based on your last period could be up to a month out. At your 12-week scan this date might be revised, and do remember less than 5 per cent of babies are born on their due dates – it's just an estimation.

A positive result

If your pregnancy test is positive, you can be pretty sure that you are in fact pregnant and don't need to do any other tests to confirm this. I had a woman jubilantly tell me that she knew she was pregnant because she'd done 20 tests just to make sure. In fact 19 of those tests were a total waste of money as, generally speaking, there is no such thing as a false positive. (A false negative is still possible, so if you test negative, you might test again a few days later and have been pregnant all along.)

 ## Lifestyle changes

As soon as you find out you're pregnant you should think carefully about how healthy your lifestyle is. As there is so much going on developmentally in the early stage, we recommend that you be particularly careful in the first 12 weeks. (After this time your fetus will be fully formed – although tiny.) The most important things to do at this stage are:

● **Stop smoking:** 9 out of 10 cot deaths happen to mothers who have smoked throughout their pregnancy.

- **Stop drinking** alcohol or taking any recreational drugs.
- **Check any meds:** If you are taking any medication, including supplements or over-the-counter drugs, check immediately that they are safe to take in pregnancy and if not discuss pregnancy-friendly alternatives.
- **Eat healthily:** You're now responsible for your baby's nutrition as well as yours.
- **Start taking folic acid:** Studies have shown this dramatically reduces the risk of spinal cord abnormalities.

Ideally you should stop drinking alcohol and smoking altogether. You should also be aware of what foods are safe to eat in pregnancy (see page 21) and try to eat a healthy balanced diet.

You will probably feel quite tired in this first trimester and, considering what your body is doing in these weeks, it's no surprise. Try to lie down if you feel really tired; you will reap the rewards. It's fine to continue exercising now, in fact it's good for you and your embryo, but don't push yourself too hard. See page 39 for more on exercising while pregnant.

Q&A

'I had a big night out before I found out I was pregnant. Will I have harmed our baby?'

We see many women who unexpectedly find out they're pregnant and are then racked with guilt because they got drunk or smoked before they knew they were pregnant. Please don't dwell on this – what has happened is in the past and there's nothing you can do about it; don't let it keep you awake. There has to be a reason we don't find out we're pregnant until two weeks after conception. Studies have shown that actually the most development takes place between 6 and 12 weeks, so, if you look after yourself at this stage, chances are you're being a good, responsible mother. In addition, implantation (the stage at which the embryo actually physically attaches to the mother) takes place about two weeks after fertilisation and, until this time, what the mother ingests is unlikely to affect the developing embryo. What it might do is prevent implantation leading to early miscarriage but, if the pregnancy continues, unwittingly drinking alcohol or smoking before you have missed your first period is unlikely to have done harm.

4 You and your baby in *the first month* (Weeks 1–4)

Most women only find out they are pregnant after the first month, when they are into their fifth or sixth week and find they have missed a period. However, some women find that the moment they conceive something changes and they may well suspect that they are pregnant.

 ## How you may be feeling
- Having tender breasts that are probably already growing
- Being surprisingly tired
- Having mood changes
- Needing to pee a lot
- Feeling nausea, with or without vomiting
- Having appetite changes – perhaps hunger, aversion to certain foods or cravings

Not all women who are pregnant will feel these symptoms; you might well feel totally normal and a positive pregnancy test might come as the biggest surprise in the world!

 ## Pregnancy tests
Pregnancy tests are becoming more and more accurate at diagnosing pregnancy before a missed period, so if you've got a suspicion that something is up, you can test a week or so before your period is due. Remember, though, that the earlier you test, the less likely it is able to detect pregnancy, so if you test negative a week before your period is due, you still have a good chance of being pregnant.

 ## Your baby
By four weeks, the embryo (actually only two weeks old) looks a bit like a tadpole but much smaller – about the size of half a grain of rice. She has already developed a vague head shape and a basic heart that is beginning to pump.

5 Nutrition in *pregnancy*

When you're suddenly responsible for the nutrition of your unborn baby, thinking about what you eat takes on another degree of importance. There are so many myths about what you should and shouldn't be eating in pregnancy, but if you're going to avoid certain foods, it's good to know why.

Do use your instinct and proceed with caution. Food poisoning is no fun at the best of times, and if you catch it when you're pregnant it will make you more unwell and therefore could affect your baby. If you're unsure about how fresh any food is, it's best to avoid it. Food hygiene is especially important in pregnancy so do be vigilant about washing fruit, vegetables and especially salad very thoroughly.

TIP *Use your common sense. As with any food, if something looks dubious, hold back.*

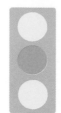

Foods to avoid

Raw shellfish (e.g. oysters)
Very high risk of food poisoning

Soft blue cheeses
Risk of listeria

Raw eggs (particularly homemade mayonnaise, homemade ice cream or chocolate mousse)
Salmonella risk

Raw meat, such as steak tartare or 'rare' steak
Listeria risk and toxoplasmosis risk

Unpasteurised milk or cheese including goat's milk or goat's cheese
Toxoplasmosis/TB risks

Pâté
Listeria risk

Liver
Contains high levels of vitamin A, which is not good in pregnancy as too much can, in rare cases, cause congenital abnormalities

Fish such as shark, marlin and swordfish
High mercury levels – which can harm your baby's nervous system

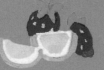

Foods to eat with caution

Tuna (fresh or tinned)
Mercury, limit consumption to two portions a week

Unwashed salad
Toxoplasmosis/listeria risk. Ensure all salad is thoroughly washed before eating

Oily fish, e.g. mackerel (also fish-oil supplements or vitamin supplements containing vitamin A)
High levels of pollutants. Limit to two portions a week

Soft cheese
Risk of listeria. If uncooked it can cause listeriosis; however, you can eat it if it is cooked – look for a good baked Camembert recipe!

Caffeine
Too much caffeine in pregnancy has been linked to miscarriage and babies with low birth weights. It is considered safe to have about 200mg a day of caffeine (2 cups of instant coffee, 3-4 mugs of tea or 200 g/7 oz of dark chocolate). Don't worry if you occasionally go over this – the risks are small – but if you regularly have more then it's worth trying to cut down

Cured meat
It was previously thought that cured meat may cause listeria but incidence is extremely low. Some cured meat has previously been cooked and any harmful bacteria destroyed. In Spain pregnant women are actively advised to eat cured ham for its health benefits! However, to be on the safe side, just freeze the cured meat for four days at home before you eat it

Foods that are (surprisingly) safe to eat

Smoked fish including smoked salmon and smoked trout

Sushi or any raw fish that has been frozen (most fish has been frozen on the boat on which it is caught. Food safety regulations require any fish used to make sushi to be frozen to -20°C (-4°F) for 24 hours before being used)

Any hard cheese, including hard blue cheeses

Soft cheese that has been pasteurised or cooked (e.g. baked Camembert)

Nuts, including peanuts, are safe to eat in pregnancy unless you are allergic to them

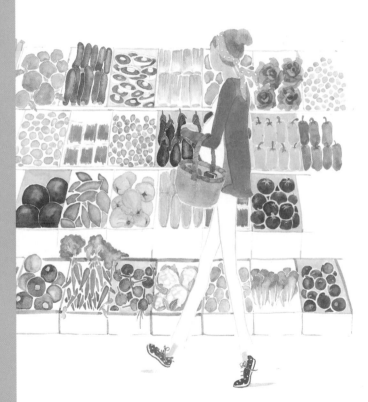

★ What you should eat

Use your pregnancy as an opportunity to eat a balanced diet. This should ideally continue once your baby is born – and is arguably more important. Children inherit food habits from their parents and, if they're brought up in a household with plenty of fruit and vegetables and having three sensible and nutritious meals a day, they're much more likely to grow into adults who embrace a healthy diet. That said, if you're really craving some junk food, it's okay to indulge yourself occasionally, just as long as you get the good stuff in.

As your bump gets bigger, it will start affecting your stomach and you'll find you have to eat little and often. It's a good idea to get into the habit of having healthy snacks, such as fruit, muesli bars and crackers, with you in case you start becoming light-headed – much better than defaulting to a chocolate bar.

Drinking during pregnancy

The Department of Health's advice is to avoid alcohol throughout pregnancy. However, research has shown that 'light drinking' – classified as one or two small glasses of wine once or twice a week – does not harm your baby. Due to the rapid development in the first trimester, it's best to avoid alcohol in the first 12 weeks of pregnancy.

★ Cravings

For many women, the onset of extraordinary cravings is the first sign they're pregnant. These can range from normal foodstuffs like spicy and salty things to extraordinary non-foods like sponges. No one really knows why pregnant women crave certain things, but as long as your cravings are not harmful and eaten in moderation, as part of a balanced diet, there's no reason why you shouldn't indulge.

Common Cravings

- Ice
- Chillies
- Gherkins
- Fruit
- Curry
- Chocolate

And the downright extraordinary ...

- Toothpaste
- Coal
- Paper
- Sponges
- Soap

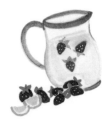

How much weight should I gain during pregnancy?

The average weight gain in pregnancy is 13.8 kg (30 lb, or 2 st 2 lb). This is broken down into the following:

Baby	3.6 kg (8 lb)
Placenta	675 g (1 lb)
Amniotic fluid	900 g (2 lb)
Growth of uterus	900 g (2 lb)
Increased breast tissue	900 g (2 lb)
Increased blood volume	1.8 kg (4 lb)
Fluid retention in mother's tissues	1.8 kg (4 lb)
Increased maternal fat stores	3.2 kg (7 lb)

The approximate weight gain per trimester is:

1st trimester: 3 kg (7 lb)
2nd trimester: 6.5 kg (14 lb)
3rd trimester: 4.5 kg (10 lb) (more in months 7–8 and less in the final month).

This differs from woman to woman, and weight gain will fluctuate from week to week. Remember these are guidelines only. People who are underweight to start with should put on more weight; those who are overweight should gain less. Tall people generally put on more weight than small people, and those whose breasts decide to expand more than the usual two cup sizes can attribute extra weight gain to this! A woman of normal weight should expect to gain between 11 and 16 kg.

'How much extra should I eat?'

Eat healthily and you won't need to eat a lot more than you normally would. There is certainly no need to 'eat for two'. In fact you only need to consume about 100 extra calories a day. By all means eat if you are hungry but make it healthy and don't let being pregnant give you the green light to binge on junk food or generally eat more than your body and your baby need – most mothers regret it when they do.

6 Early *miscarriage*

As exciting as it is to find out that you are pregnant, you should bear in mind that before 12 weeks there is a relatively high chance of miscarriage. Exact figures are hard to come by, but it's estimated that up to one in every three to four pregnancies ends in miscarriage. This decreases as you near 12 weeks. The most common symptoms of miscarriage are bleeding and severe cramping, but these symptoms do not necessarily mean you are miscarrying. If you have any bleeding, speak to your doctor and they will arrange a scan. Some people miscarry without there being any outward signs. This is called a 'missed miscarriage' and will often only be detected on a scan. Please try not to spend your first trimester obsessing about miscarriage; if you're feeling rotten, these pregnancy symptoms are often a really good sign that your pregnancy is progressing nicely.

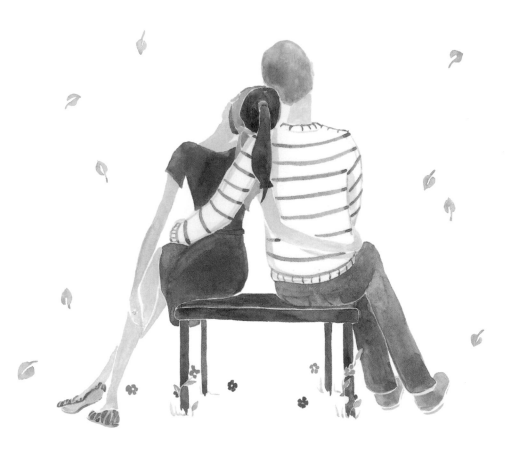

> *'I found out at 12 weeks that I'd had a missed miscarriage and I was beside myself. I had no idea that if I hadn't had a bleed that I could have had a miscarriage. Dealing with the news was hard and people react in different ways. The one thing that really stuck with me was my father-in-law saying, "Well, we know your body works perfectly. You got pregnant, but your body also knew when the baby wasn't meant to be." The macabre rationale really resounded with me. I got pregnant six months later and my son is perfect. In a funny way, I'm glad that I had a miscarriage because if I hadn't, I wouldn't have Ludo.'* MARINA

The reason people often wait until after their 12-week check to tell all their friends and to start getting excited about their pregnancy, is because of this high chance of miscarriage. That said, don't feel you have to keep your pregnancy entirely to yourself. There are some people that will be a valuable support if you do need them. As a general guide, we advise people to tell those friends and family whom they would want to talk to if they did have a miscarriage.

If you do have a miscarriage, be prepared: it is emotional and often the feelings can hit you later than you expect. Often there is no reason why it happens, and you just have to accept that miscarriage is very natural. You could see it as nature's way of preventing mothers having to take a difficult decision at 12 or even 20 weeks if they discover their fetus has a severe abnormality that is not compatible with life. For most women, having a miscarriage will not preclude them from having children in the near future. Some women suffer from recurrent miscarriage – if this is the case, there are medical interventions that will hopefully enable you to have children. If you have any questions or worries, do talk to your doctor, but above all try to remember that it's a lot more common than most people realise and talked about less than it should be.

7 You and your baby in the *second month* (Weeks 5–8)

Once you've had the confirmation that you're pregnant, you should make an appointment to see your GP, who will discuss antenatal care, looking after yourself in pregnancy and any other concerns you may have.

 ### How you may be feeling

The symptoms described in the first month are likely to continue, and there could be some additional nausea, flatulence, constipation, headaches and increased vaginal discharge to throw into the mix! You may also notice skin changes and the beginnings of varicose veins.

Early scans

From around six weeks it is possible to detect the embryo on a scan. Early scans are not routine on the NHS (unless there have been complications) but it is possible to get it done privately if you want. Early scans will check the following:

- Whether the embryo has a heartbeat.
- If the embryo has implanted in the correct place, inside the uterus. (Rarely the embryo implants outside the uterus. This is called an ectopic pregnancy, and it means that not only is the pregnancy not viable but that urgent treatment is needed for the safety of the mother.)
- How many embryos you are carrying.

The early scan is often an internal scan, where the ultrasound probe is inserted into the vagina. This gives the sonographer a better view. It is painless and discreet but something you and your partner should be prepared for.

Your baby

The embryo is now about the size of a raspberry, and the little tail that it had has now gone. Arms and legs have formed and these are moving a lot, although you won't be able to feel it yet. At eight weeks, the embryo weighs about a gram, already has a little tongue and is busy developing taste buds.

> *'In spite of how miserable they make me feel, I've always been reassured by rotten early pregnancy symptoms. With my first pregnancy, I had not an ounce of sickness and when those in the know asked me how I was feeling I delightedly told them that I was fine and, in fact, I didn't even feel pregnant. Those words came back to haunt me when, at my 12-week scan, there was no heartbeat; my lack of symptoms was a sign that all was not well. With my subsequent pregnancies, I've always sought solace in the extreme fatigue and nausea rather than feel sorry for myself. This is not to say that alarm bells should ring if you don't have any nausea; there are many women who sail through their pregnancy feeling even better than usual.'* MARINA

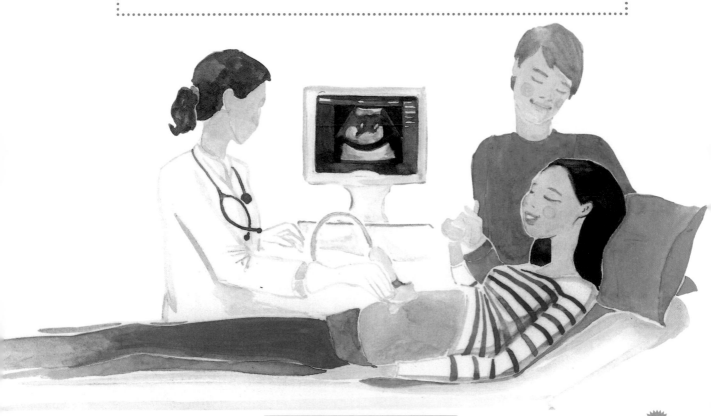

8 Morning *sickness*

Morning – or what often turns out to be all-day – sickness, is a real pain. Just at the point where they're nervously excited about their pregnancy, but reluctant to let people know about it, around 80 per cent of women are struck down with nausea often compounded by extreme tiredness. The degree to which women experience morning sickness varies greatly: some don't feel a thing, while others are placed on a drip in hospital because they're unable to keep anything inside them.

Morning sickness usually hits hardest between weeks 4 and 12 of pregnancy – exactly at the time when the crucial development is happening in the fetus. A lot of women become despondent and depressed after weeks of feeling atrocious and so it's important to keep your spirits up. No one really knows why morning sickness occurs, but because it's happening just when all the most crucial developments are taking place, it's a good sign that your pregnancy is progressing well.

 ## When morning sickness is more severe

If you are finding that you are really not coping with the nausea and/or you are vomiting so much that you really can't keep much inside (a condition known as 'hyperemesis gravidarum'), then it is time to seek medical advice. This is usually in the form of oral anti-nausea medication or, if severe, hospitalisation for this medication to be put directly into the veins along with some intravenous fluid.

There is always a balance of weighing risk against benefit, and this is something that mothers (and doctors) constantly need to do in pregnancy. In this case, the (small) risk to the baby in taking the medication is outweighed by the increased risk to the baby if the mother is so unwell she becomes dehydrated, malnourished and overtired. Although the medications have not undergone formal trials in pregnant women (as it is difficult and often unethical to do good clinical trials on pregnant women), they have been widely used in pregnancy for decades and have been found to be safe.

 ## How to cope with morning sickness

Everyone wants to know how to alleviate morning sickness and, unfortunately, there is no clinically proven natural cure. We do, however, talk to the many Bump Class girls about what worked for them and have found that there is anecdotal evidence that the ideas opposite might work.

Eat little and often: Your body is working so hard in the first trimester, it needs energy to sustain this. While officially we're told that pregnant women only need to consume around 100 or so more calories per day while pregnant, it might be that you need to exceed that and eat more frequently, just for the first trimester. Try to get into the habit of having a healthy snack on you at all times. A lot of women find hunger leads very quickly to nausea, so if you can have a quick snack when that first hunger pang develops, you might be able to stave off the nausea.

Combat nausea with eating: Although you might not feel like eating anything while you're feeling sick, eating often helps with the sickness. Most pregnant women prefer bland, starchy foods like *toast* and *crackers*.

Make sure you are drinking enough: If you find water boring, try adding some sliced *lemon, orange, mint* or *cucumber*; it will make it taste much better. Also try to drink *herbal tea.*

Try ginger: It is a natural anti-emetic so *ginger tea* or *biscuits* can help with the nausea. It doesn't matter if it is fresh – just try to include ginger in your diet where you can tolerate it.

Some studies have shown that vitamin B12 can help with morning sickness. Its highest concentration is found in liver (which unfortunately is not recommended in pregnancy) and shellfish (which should only be eaten if cooked). It is also found in *fish, cheese* and *eggs*. If you can't stomach these, try using a supplement instead.

Amazingly enough, a lot of girls report that doing a little bit of exercise often kicks that interminable feeling of nausea. It's the last thing you'll feel like doing but it's amazing what a brisk walk or a quick 20 minutes on a cross-trainer will do for you.

Sleep and rest seem to correlate directly to morning sickness; after a bad night's sleep, women often report feeling sicker. Try to have a rest during the day – you're not being lazy, your body is doing so much in this early stage and it's crucial you get more sleep than you usually need.

Acupuncture and reflexology can be really helpful in treating a whole host of common, normal but annoying pregnancy symptoms. Although the evidence behind them is not concrete, many mothers have found that complementary techniques have helped them through their pregnancy. Make sure you see someone who has a knowledge of pregnancy and the right qualifications but most of all who you trust – more often than not this can make all the difference.

Stay positive: This is often easier said than done but your state of mind will often have a huge bearing on how you feel. We promise that this is all worthwhile for the years of joy your baby will bring you!

9 Other early *pregnancy symptoms*

As if nausea and vomiting weren't enough for newly pregnant women to contend with, early pregnancy often presents a whole host of new and unexpected symptoms. The first three months are commonly considered the most difficult of pregnancy, often with debilitating symptoms, but as this is when the majority of fetal development occurs, it is better to avoid medication if possible.

⭐ Breast tenderness
This is often the first sign that women have that they are pregnant and is a reassuring sign that the pregnancy is going well. For most people it is not debilitating, but if it is, hot water bottles or warm flannels can ease the symptoms or, failing that, paracetamol is considered to be a safe and effective painkiller to take during pregnancy.

⭐ Frequent urination
Somewhat surprisingly this is a problem for many women in the first three months of pregnancy as much as towards the end. The drastic hormone changes mean that many women suddenly need to run to the loo several times a night and more often during the day. You will probably find that you are drinking more water as well. If you are finding the night-time calls of nature a problem, then cutting back on the fluid you drink in the evening can help. Just make sure you make up for it in the day.

⭐ Constipation
The bowels do tend to become somewhat sluggish in pregnancy, and the best way to deal with this particular problem is to increase the amount of fibre in your diet and to drink plenty of water. Prune juice, kiwis and dried fruit are all good natural ways to speed transit!

⭐ Fatigue
It is common to feel extraordinarily tired in the first trimester of pregnancy and really that is your body telling you to rest as it needs the extra energy to make the baby! Listen to your body and try to go to bed early – and if possible catch a few winks during the day too.

⭐ Vaginal discharge
Many pregnant women find that their normal vaginal discharge changes during pregnancy. It is common for the amount to increase and for it to be of a more watery consistency. If there

are any other symptoms like a change in smell or an itch or pain, make sure you see your doctor to check that there is no infection. If you have any bleeding during pregnancy you should see your doctor. Although it does not necessarily mean that there is a problem, it always needs to be checked out.

 Other possible symptoms

There are lots of other pregnancy symptoms that you will hear people talk about. It has been hypothesised that the symptoms you suffer from in pregnancy are often the ones that may plague you in old age, so this can serve as an early warning to look after that particular aspect of your health sooner rather than later!

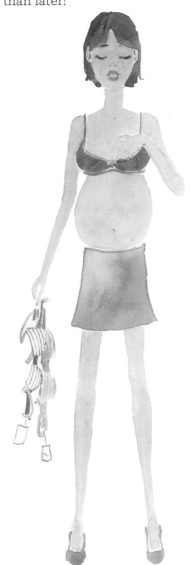

Here are a few of the other symptoms people commonly note:
- Worsening of eczema
- Worsening of asthma
- Joint pain
- Bloating
- Abdominal cramps
- Itchy skin
- Thrush

Useful things to have on you:
- Dry biscuits
- Dried fruit/nuts
- Muesli bars
- Herbal tea bags
- Ginger biscuits
- Small bottle of water
- Mints
- Panty liners
- Paracetamol
- Access to a loo ...

10 Your birth *options*

As soon as you know you're pregnant, it's worth thinking about your options when it comes to giving birth. A generation ago, everyone went to hospital, but nowadays there is a range of options to give mothers the best possible experience, both within the NHS and privately. Remember, it's rarely too late to change your mind, although sometimes this can be a hassle.

When you find out you're pregnant, you need to speak to your GP to register with the hospital you would like to give birth at. It's worth doing a bit of research to make sure they have the facilities that you want, but consider booking somewhere near to home. However, what a lot of people don't realise is that there are options within the NHS.

	Pro's	Cons
Labour ward This is the traditional place where women give birth – essentially at the hospital.	Once you're in established labour you'll be given your own room and one-to-one midwife care. Doctors and anaesthetists are on hand if you need them. Should something go wrong and either you or your baby need medical help, you're in the best place.	Hospitals can sometimes be quite intimidating environments, and not being relaxed and comfortable can slow down the labour. Because the NHS is entirely free of charge, the staff and resources are understandably stretched. They will make the safety of you and your baby an absolute priority, but not necessarily your comfort – not because they don't care, but because they have limited resources. Once your baby is born, you will be transferred to the postnatal ward, which can sometimes be slightly chaotic.

	Pro's	Cons
Birth centre attached to a hospital There are an increasing amount of midwife-led birth centres attached to major NHS hospitals.	Birth centres attached to hospitals are wonderful places to give birth as they provide the homely midwife-led environment that labouring women tend to thrive in, while being attached to major hospitals should emergency care be needed.	As birth centres are midwife-led, they are unable to administer any medical pain relief such as an epidural. However, since they're attached to a hospital, women can easily be transferred to the labour ward in the hospital for this to happen. If you're deemed high risk, you may not be allowed to give birth in a birth centre.
Stand-alone birth centre These are free-standing midwife-led units that are not attached to a hospital per se.	As with birth centres attached to hospitals, women benefit from the 'home from home' environment.	For first-time mothers, the likelihood that they will need to be transferred to a hospital is relatively high (36–45 per cent). If you're seriously considering a free-standing birth centre, think about it practically. Especially for first-time mothers, the proximity to a hospital is more important than the view from the birth pool. Again, if you're considered high risk, you may not be able to give birth in one of these centres.
Home birth If you wish, the NHS will support you and provide midwife-led care in order for you to have a home birth. The midwives will perform your antenatal checks and a midwife team will arrive to deliver your baby.	Studies have shown that women who are relaxed in their environment, particularly in their own homes, have easier labours with less need for medical intervention. The same midwife team will care for you throughout your pregnancy and will deliver your baby so you will benefit from the continuity of care that has been shown to be beneficial to women.	Studies have shown that home births are slightly higher risk than births at hospitals or their attached birth centre for first-time mothers. Should you or your baby require urgent medical attention, you will have to get to hospital. Although extreme cases are rare, it's worth considering your proximity to hospital. If you're deemed high risk, you will be discouraged from having a home birth for the sake of your baby and yourself.

11 What care you can expect in your *pregnancy*

The NHS makes us proud to be British. In spite of its imperfections, it provides comprehensive care for pregnant women from the beginning of their pregnancy, through their labour and recovery and after their baby has been born, and it is entirely free of charge as long as you're a UK resident.

The timings of your various tests and checks may vary, but below is a timeline showing roughly when you will see your doctor or midwife during your pregnancy.

As well as the key scans at 12 weeks and 20 weeks you will have regular standard checks, usually performed by a midwife, which increase in regularity as you near your due date. If your midwife is at all concerned about you or your baby, or you're deemed high risk, you will be seen by a doctor. You may not see a doctor at all during your pregnancy if your pregnancy is uncomplicated, and that is absolutely fine.

> **Standard checks**
> Measure the uterus, check the baby's position and heart rate, and check your blood pressure and urine.

8–12 weeks	**Booking appointment:** This is the very first appointment with a midwife or GP and usually happens at 8–12 weeks. See page 48 for further details on this.
10–12 weeks	You can choose to have a NIPT (non-invasive prenatal test) at this point if you like, although this is not currently available on the NHS (see page 50).
12-week (nuchal) scan and check-up	If you're deemed low risk and your pregnancy is uncomplicated, you will be offered an ultrasound scan at around 12 weeks as well as a blood test to calculate the risk of major chromosomal abnormalities such as Down's syndrome. See page 50 for more information on this important scan.
16-week check-up	Here you will have the results of the 12-week blood tests and ultrasound scan. The midwife will check your blood pressure and urine and discuss any concerns you have.

20-week (anomaly) scan	This is an important ultrasound scan that checks that your fetus is developing as it should. See page 72 for more on this.
25-week check-up	This is only done with first pregnancies. The midwife will do the standard checks.
28-week check-up	The standard checks will be done and there might be a glucose tolerance test to check for gestational diabetes. If you are rhesus negative (see page 49) you will probably have your first anti-D injection at this point.
31-week check-up	Only done in first pregnancies, the results of the glucose test are discussed, and the standard checks are done.

It's not uncommon for women in their third trimester to develop anaemia, an iron deficiency which makes you feel tired. If this is the case, mention it to your midwife who may suggest a blood test and iron supplements.

34-week check-up	The birth plan is discussed and the standard checks are done. If you are rhesus negative you will probably have your second anti-D treatment.

If there are any concerns about your baby's well-being, growth or position, you should be offered a late scan in the third trimester. If there aren't specific concerns but you want some reassurance, or you simply want to see your baby, you can pay for a private scan.

36-week check-up	The standard checks are done.
38-week check-up	Here the midwife or GP will discuss going overdue and will do the standard checks.
40-week check-up	This is only for a first baby. The standard checks are done.
41-week check-up	The standard checks are done and the midwife or GP will also offer a membrane sweep and discuss options for induction (see page 114).

If you choose to have your baby privately, you will be seen slightly more frequently and will have more scans. However, if you are being looked after in the NHS it is absolutely fine to supplement your care with some additional privately paid scans. You might want to have an early viability scan at six to eight weeks and a third trimester fetal growth and well-being scan at around 34 weeks.

You might also want to pay for a Group B Strep screen late in your pregnancy. This tests for the bacteria Group B Streptococcus, which could potentially cause infection (see page 129). The NHS do not routinely screen for this, but you can send off for a postal service for around £35 (see www.tdlpathology.com for testing and further information).

Q&A

'Why do I need all these urine tests?'

As you progress through your pregnancy, you might get a little tired of all the urine tests. They are really important as they are used to detect protein in the urine, which, in combination with blood-pressure measurements, can be a sign of pre-eclampsia, a dangerous condition that can affect pregnant women towards the end of pregnancy. If not treated it can lead to eclampsia, which can cause seizures in the mother and, although rare, can result in maternal death. Signs to watch out for are: a headache, pain in the top of your tummy, excessive swelling (particularly of face, hands and feet), visual disturbance (double vision or flashing lights) or vomiting. The test will also screen for urine infections, which are more common in pregnancy.

Some first-time mothers feel that they don't get seen quite as often as they might expect in the first couple of trimesters. Remember though, your care plan has been carefully worked out and if they need to see you more they will. In the final trimester your check-ups and monitoring will increase. Don't forget, you can always speak to the team looking after you if you have any concerns at any point in your pregnancy.

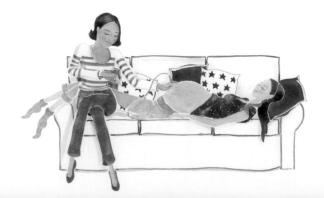

12 Exercise in *pregnancy*

Labour is often compared to running a marathon and, if you look at your pregnancy as like preparing for that marathon, fitness and strength are key. But it's not only labour that you need to be strong for: as you get heavier in pregnancy you need to be stronger, and then, once your baby is born, carrying her, holding her and hoicking her and the endless gear she needs around requires the strength of an athlete. New mothers often put fitness at the bottom of their inevitably long list of 'things to do' and as a result it gets overlooked. In fact it should be at the top; a healthy, strong mother who can cope with the physical toll of motherhood will be a better mother to her baby.

 How hard should I exercise?
Your level of exercise in pregnancy depends on your fitness before you got pregnant. As a rule, aim to do about 80 per cent of what you were doing before you were pregnant at the beginning of your pregnancy and adjust this as your pregnancy progresses.

Every person's body is individual, and how hard you exercise depends on your fitness and build. Always trust your instinct; if you feel like something is not doing you any good or becomes painful, then stop and do something different.

Generally your heart rate should not go above 140 beats per minute. As we don't tend to wear heart rate monitors on a daily basis, this can be tough to determine, so, as a rule of thumb, you should always be able to have a conversation with someone while you're exercising.

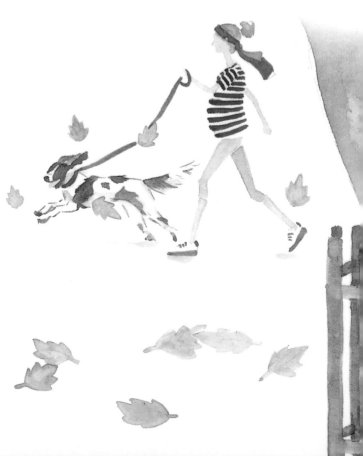

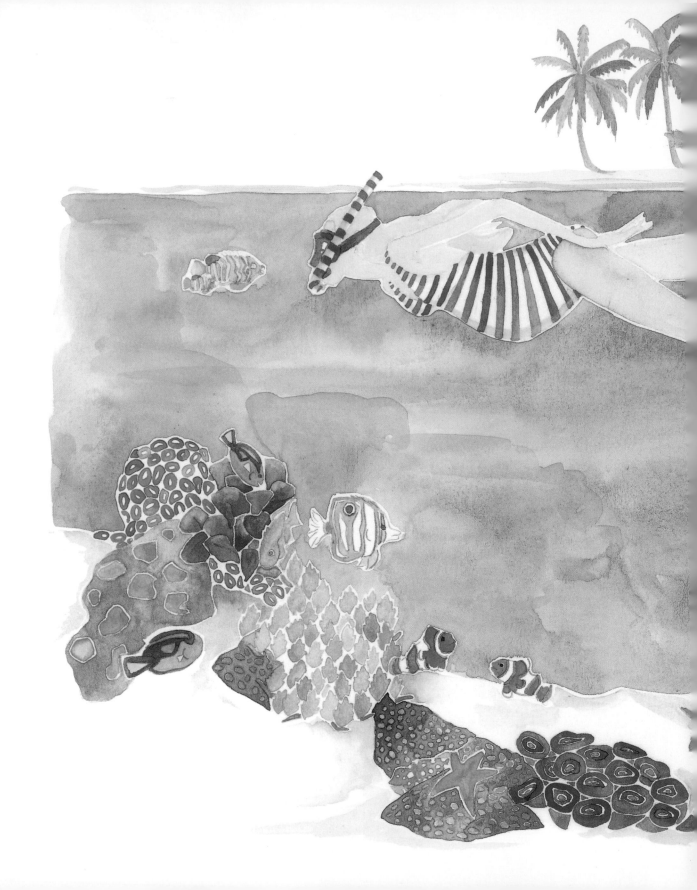

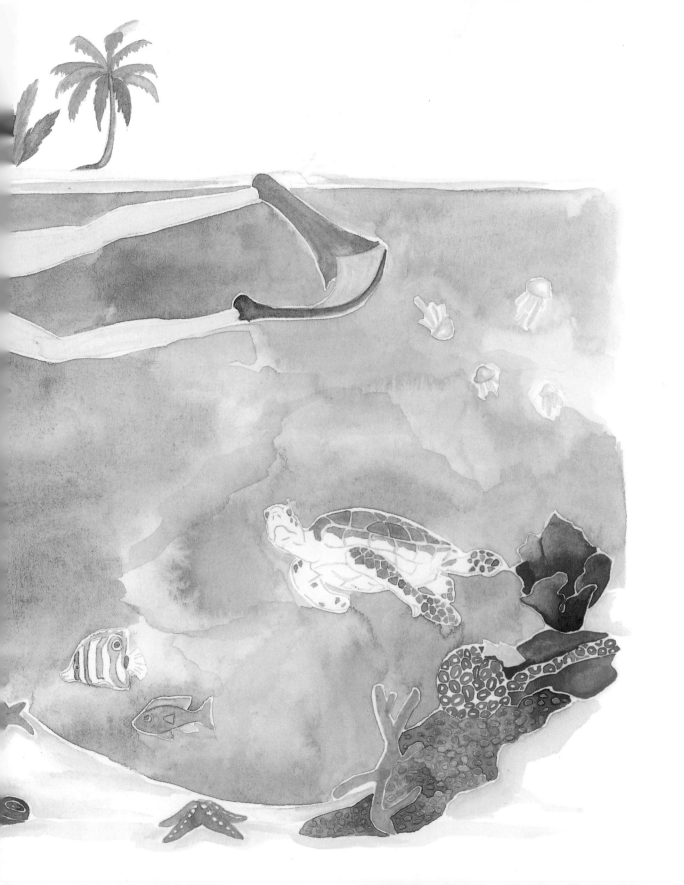

What exercise to avoid during pregnancy

- Contact sports
- Sports with a risk of falling – e.g. skiing, horse riding or cycling
- Scuba diving
- High-impact sports that you are not used to – e.g. running if you did not run regularly before
- Power Plate machines
- Exercises that involve you lying on your back (after 16 weeks)

Be cautious: from about week 8 your body releases a hormone called relaxin which essentially makes your muscles, joints and ligaments more supple, allowing your body to accommodate your growing baby. It does, however, also put you at more risk of injury so don't push yourself too hard. If you feel anything unusual while you're exercising, don't stop suddenly as this can make you feel quite faint. Instead, spend a few minutes walking around and if symptoms continue or you're worried speak to your midwife.

'If something is hurting, stop doing whatever is making it hurt. Acute pain is your body's way of telling you to stop. I see too many women trying to endure the pain, which just makes things worse. If the pain persists, go and see a women's health physiotherapist.'
CAMILLA LAWRENCE, WOMEN'S HEATH PHYSIOTHERAPIST AT THE BUMP CLASS

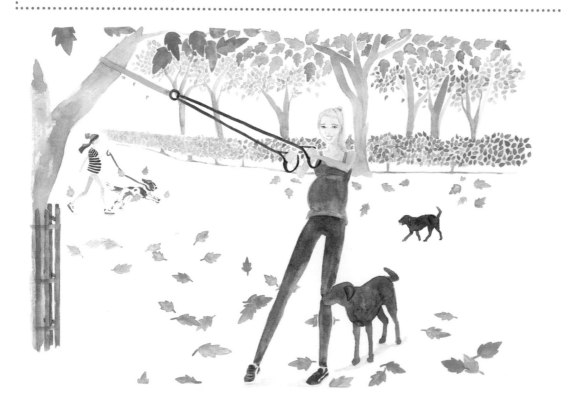

First trimester

Unless you've been advised to cut out sports by your doctor there is no reason for you not to continue with what you were doing before you found out you were pregnant, using the 80 per cent rule. Many people suffering from morning sickness find that a gentle workout eases their nausea. If you haven't been exercising then you should think about starting. Start gently and gradually build up your fitness. Remember that any exercise you manage to fit in will be beneficial for you in the long term. Ideally combine cardio and some strength-conditioning work five times a week, but if all you can manage is one session a week, your time will not have been wasted.

Second trimester

As your bump starts to grow, this is the time to stop pushing yourself too hard. Look into antenatal exercise classes that will take into account the strains your body is under. Antenatal yoga, Pilates and barre-core (ballet-style exercises) are great at strength building, but make sure you also fit in some cardiovascular exercise such as swimming, static cycling, using a cross-trainer or even just having a brisk walk a few times a week.

Third trimester

This is the trimester where you'll notice how much growing your baby does and this does make exercise harder. Try to make time in your day as you will reap the rewards, but your routine might have to be altered slightly. Women in their third trimester often love swimming – it's a great way to get some cardiovascular exercise in without straining your joints, and the feeling of relative weightlessness is welcome respite.

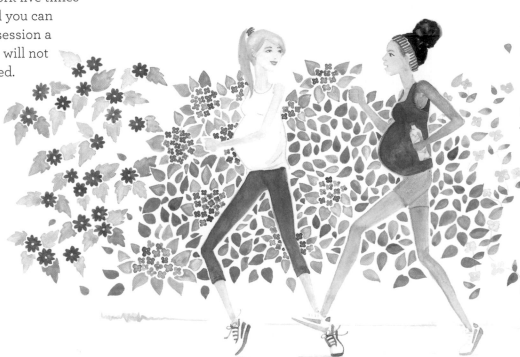

13 Pelvic floor *exercises*

Possibly one of the most important things to do in pregnancy is exercising your pelvic floor. In an ideal world, all women would do this for their whole lives, but it's especially important in pregnancy because these muscles are under particular strain during your pregnancy and then through labour.

Your pelvic floor is a hammock of muscles that run under the pelvis connecting the pubic bone at the front to the coccyx at the back. These muscles support your bladder, bowel, uterus and reproductive organs as well as the joints of your pelvis. They also wrap around the urethra, rectum and vagina, making them crucial in keeping women continent and sexually sensitive.

For generations, women were led to believe that incontinence was just part of being a mother. This is not the case, and incontinence, while common, is not normal: regular pelvic floor exercises can completely prevent this.

To contract your pelvic floor imagine you are trying to stop your flow of urine and stop passing wind at the same time – you should feel a squeeze and lift in the muscles underneath you. Nothing else should move, in fact the joy is that you can do these exercises wherever you are; no one will be any the wiser.

 How to do pelvic floor exercises
You should be doing two types of exercise:
1) **Slow:** While gently breathing, squeeze and hold your pelvic floor for as long as you can for up to 10 seconds and then relax completely. The gold standard is 10 repetitions of 10-second holds, but many pregnant women will not achieve this. Don't worry: with practice, you will. You need to make sure you actually feel a release at the end of each squeeze. If not, you've probably released earlier; there's no point in counting to 10 if you've actually released at 5.

2) **Fast:** Squeeze your pelvic floor strongly and immediately let go again. Repeat 10 times. The release is as important as the squeeze so make sure you are releasing properly, rather than only halfway.

Ideally you should try to do a set of slow and fast squeezes three to six times a day. You should not be clenching your buttocks or moving your legs or back while making any movements.

The difficulty for most is not doing the exercises, but *remembering* to do them. Try to think of things you do daily that will remind you to do them, for instance brushing your teeth or sitting at a red traffic light. You can do them in any position – lying, sitting or standing. You can even do them walking, although this is more challenging!

It's just as important to do your pelvic floor exercises if you're having a caesarean. Studies have shown that for the majority of women the pelvic floor is mostly weakened by carrying a baby for nine months rather than a vaginal delivery.

Once you've got used to these exercises, you should push yourself to hold the long ones for longer and increase the number of repetitions you do in a set. Try to spread the exercises out during the day – you can do them at any time (except when passing urine). Try to engage your pelvic floor during the day when you cough, sneeze or lift. Developing this habit will stand you in great stead for the rest of your life.

'I really struggled to remember to do my pelvic floor exercises so I decided to put six pens in a special pot on my desk at work. During the day, every time I did a set of exercises I'd put one of my pens back into the main pot, and by the end of the day, those pens need to be cleared. No one knew the significance of my pens or even that I was furiously exercising my pelvic floor. I've always liked multi-tasking!' VANESSA, THE BUMP CLASS

For some women, the idea of contracting these muscles is totally alien or they have no idea whether or not they are doing them right. If you're in doubt (and it is worth getting this right) or you're having problems with even mild incontinence, go and see a women's health physiotherapist – they will test the strength of your pelvic floor and make sure you're doing everything correctly!

'If I really work on strengthening my pelvic floor, won't it make it harder for my baby to come out?'
This is something we get asked a lot on the Bump Class, and the answer is a definite no. Camilla Lawrence, our women's health physiotherapist, advises that exercising your pelvic floor will not make those muscles shorter or tighter, just more powerful – like when you exercise any muscle in the body. The pelvic floor muscles will still be able to fully relax and stretch as normal. Numerous research studies have shown that doing regular pelvic floor exercises in pregnancy will have no adverse effects on your labour.

14 Looking after yourself *physically*

Adjusting to motherhood is challenging for any woman, and dealing with pain from an injury sustained while you were pregnant is something all women can do without. Here are a few pointers that, if heeded, should help your body cope with the physical rigours of pregnancy.

- Engage your abdominal muscles. Bump Class physio, Camilla Lawrence, advises: 'Don't let it all hang out just because you're pregnant. Your tummy muscles are a corset, providing the structure that supports your body, and if there's ever a time they need to be strong, it's when you're pregnant.'
- Try not to stand for long periods of time, especially when you reach your second trimester. When you are standing, stand tall and gently engage your tummy muscles. High heels exacerbate all these pressures, so avoid wearing them.
- Try not to lie on your back from around 20 weeks, either when resting or exercising. As your baby grows your uterus becomes significantly heavier. When lying down, this will put pressure on a crucial blood vessel called the vena cava and can restrict the blood flow. If this happens you will feel the effects well before your baby will. You will instantly feel very uncomfortable and unwell (usually nauseous and short of breath), and you will instinctively move. So, if you wake up and you're on your back, don't worry; your baby's well-being will not have been compromised.
- As they get larger, pregnant women start to waddle. Instead of standing tall with their core engaged, they rock from side to side, swinging each leg around, which is terrible for the back and pelvis. Ideally warn those who spend time with you to spot any waddling and remind you not to do it.
- If you can avoid doing any heavy lifting and housework in your last trimester, your body will thank you. Real killers are loading the dishwasher (especially the bottom rack) and lifting heavy objects. If you have to do these, try to engage your abdominal and pelvic floor muscles as you lift.
- Getting in and out of cars can be really hard on your back in later pregnancy. To make life easier and reduce the risk of damage, keep your legs together when getting in or out and sit on a plastic carrier bag so that you can easily swivel!
- Avoid painful activities. This is not the time for 'no pain, no gain' – if something hurts, stop doing it.
- Avoid 'abdominal doming'. Have you noticed that occasionally when under strain (for instance sitting up in the bath or bed) your tummy forms a funny kind

of dome shape? As amusing as this might be, it's actually not great for your abdominal muscles and may be causing them to strain and separate down the midline.

Tips for avoiding abdominal doming

- **Bed:** Instead of performing a giant sit-up to get up, bend your knees, keeping your knees together, and roll gently onto your side so that your knees are on the edge of the bed. Using your hands, push your body up at the same time as you let your feet down the side of the bed. Do the opposite when you get into bed.

- **Car:** Rather than the usual one-legged diagonal squat to get into the car, put a plastic bag on your car seat, stand with your back to the side of the seat and sit down. Once sitting, use your hands and feet to swivel round into the driving position. The plastic bag will make the swivel much easier and can stay there while you drive, ready for you to swivel to get back out of the car.

- **Bath:** We've known countless women get stuck in the bath while pregnant. With one hand in front of you on the side of the bath and one hand behind at the base of the bath, use your arms to pull and push yourself up into a squat position, with one leg in front of the other. Once there, take a moment to breathe before you stand up. Buy a non-slip bath mat, as this will make the bath less slippery and easier to manoeuvre yourself. A bath mat is not only useful for pregnant women but comes in really useful to stop energetic toddlers nosediving into the bath. As your pregnancy progresses, make sure you have your phone handy while in the bath. If you do get stuck, at least you can call for help.

If you're in pain, seek treatment from a specialist obstetric physiotherapist. It's not 'normal' to be in pain during pregnancy. Don't be a hero – you're more likely to be able to fix something quickly if you get it seen early.

THE BUMP CLASS

15 You and your baby in the *third month* (Weeks 9–13)

Your first antenatal appointment

As you approach week 12 you will probably have your first antenatal appointment (or booking appointment). This will probably be the longest appointment in your pregnancy. Your midwife or doctor will want to:

- Talk about your past medical and obstetric history and your general health.
- Check the date of your last period to give you an estimated date of delivery. This may change after you have had your 12-week scan, as this is now deemed to be more reliable.
- Do a physical examination.
- Do a series of blood and urine tests:
- Check blood type and rhesus status
- Urine screen for sugar, protein and infection
- Blood tests to check general health, antibody levels and immunity to certain diseases such as rubella
- Tests to exclude presence of sexually transmitted infections
- Blood sugar test
- If you are of African or Mediterranean origin you'll be offered tests for sickle-cell anaemia and thalassaemia.

 ## How you may be feeling

Having a proper bump is still a way off, although you will have probably noticed your waist starting to thicken and there might well be some clothes that no longer feel comfortable. By 12 weeks, your nausea and vomiting may be slowing down but could be replaced by headaches and dizziness.

At around 12 weeks you'll have your first routine scan (see page 50), and, if all is well, this is when most couples choose to share the exciting news.

 ## Your baby

At the beginning of the third month your embryo graduates to being a fetus and is beginning to grow very quickly. During this month the bones and cartilage are forming and the fetus is beginning to swallow. Her facial features are becoming more distinct and her heart is fully functioning and pumping

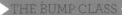

blood around her body. By 13 weeks she weighs around 23 g, is about 7–8 cm (3 inches) long and has eyes and ears, fingernails and even tooth buds. Your fetus has now done most of her development and the important systems are fully formed. From now, it's all about growing!

Concerns if you're rhesus negative

At your booking appointment they check for your blood group (either A, B, AB or O) and rhesus status (positive or negative). Both of these are determined by your genes and will not change. Most people are rhesus positive – this means you have a protein called a D antigen on your red blood cells. If you are rhesus negative, you don't.

If you are rhesus negative and your baby is rhesus positive (inherited from the father), there could be potential problems. If your baby's blood comes into contact with your blood (known as sensitisation), your body will treat it as a foreign invader and produce antibodies to fight it. The first time this happens (i.e. in a first pregnancy), it is not usually an issue. The problems arise if you have another baby who is also rhesus positive. The antibodies you made in your first pregnancy will cross the placenta and attack the baby's blood cells, which could potentially cause fetal anaemia.

Before you start to panic: this situation can easily be prevented by giving you injections of 'anti-D' at various stages during the pregnancy. This prevents your system making the antibodies against your baby. Protocol as to when and how much anti-D is given varies from place to place, and you should follow the protocol of the hospital where you will be delivering. All hospitals are obliged to test rhesus status at booking and will give you anti-D appropriately.

Being rhesus negative is really quite common (it occurs in 15 per cent of Caucasian women), so please don't worry about it. The important thing to remember is that if you have a 'sensitising event' (e.g. a fall, physical trauma, a bleed or amniocentesis or CVS – see page 245) or delivery of your baby you need to have anti-D within 72 hours. This is one of the most important reasons to always carry your notes with you!

The first opportunity we have to check if the baby is rhesus positive or negative is after she is born when blood from the umbilical cord is taken to check. If she is positive you will be given another dose of anti-D within 72 hours of the birth.

16 The 12-week check-up (nuchal scan)

The 12-week check-up is really important. Using a combination of ultrasound scanning (using jelly on the tummy – this is harmless for the fetus and mother) and a blood test, it determines the risk of the fetus having a chromosomal abnormality, such as Down's syndrome, as well as many other things, including heart defects, genetic syndromes and structural abnormalities. The ultrasound scan also checks the fetus is growing well but one of the main purposes is to look at the translucent or clear space in the tissue at the back of your fetus' neck, hence the name 'nuchal translucency scan'. Sometimes this scan is also called the 'dating scan' as it can more accurately predict the due date of your baby than dating from your last period.

In order for the tests to be accurate, the check-up must be done between 11 and 14 weeks. It does not give you a diagnosis of any abnormalities, simply an idea of whether you are at high or low risk of certain conditions. If the risk is deemed high you may be advised to have CVS (chorionic villus sampling) or amniocentesis tests (see Glossary, pages 245 and 244); these are the only 100 per cent accurate ways of testing for chromosomal abnormalities. However, they are invasive and associated with a small risk of miscarriage. Bear in mind that CVS is not usually done after 14 weeks so it is a good idea to do the 12-week scan earlier rather than later, allowing time to arrange further tests if necessary.

 Non-invasive prenatal testing (NIPT)
There is a type of screening test that detects fetal DNA in the mother's blood; however, at the time of writing it is only available privately in the UK. It involves a simple blood test from the mother, taken from 10 weeks, and gives a more accurate risk assessment for genetic abnormalities, such as Down's syndrome, than the standard screening test. There are various brand names for this test and generally they are over 99 per cent accurate – as opposed to the standard test, which is only 93 per cent accurate. It therefore decreases the risk of unnecessary invasive testing.

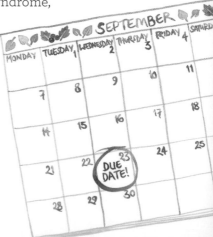

Q&A

'My due date from my scan is different from my due date from my last period. Which do I go by?'

It is now widely accepted that due dates predicted from scans are the most accurate. Of course, if you have had IVF and know the precise date of implantation, you will know exactly. If you 'know' because 'it only happened on one night', remember that sperm live for up to seven days so fertilisation can occur on the day you have sex (if you happen to ovulate that day) or a few days later.

It is fairly common for your due date to be recalculated after your scan and might have changed by up to a week or so. The scan date is more accurate but do bear in mind that your baby is likely to arrive anywhere between three weeks before and two weeks after that date.

TIPS

- It is worth thinking about and discussing with your partner your views on what actions you would take should the screening test indicate a high risk of an abnormality.
- Do remember that for the unlucky few the 12-week scan is the time they find out that they have had a miscarriage if no heartbeat is detected. This may have occurred a few weeks earlier but because there may not have been bleeding it might have gone unnoticed.
- If you have not had an early scan, the 12-week scan may also be the time you find out you are having twins!

'My friend Lizzy made the mistake of making a big thing of her due date. The well-meaning texts and phone calls started on the due date, and by the time she was 10 days overdue, these calls were driving her crazy. Already irritable and entirely fed up with being pregnant, her family and friends' concern added to her stress. When she got pregnant for the second time, Lizzy told her enthusiastic family that she was due two weeks later than she actually was. The surprise in telling them about the birth before anyone was expecting it was far more enjoyable than being besieged by anticipation.' MARINA

17 Being pregnant with *Twins or multiples*

The time most people find out they are having twins is at the first scan, at 12 weeks. If you're not expecting this, it can be quite a shock, but don't worry: you've still got a few months to prepare and get used to the idea.

Identical twins are created when one egg is fertilised and subsequently splits, so the DNA is the same in both twins. With non-identical twins, two eggs are released and fertilised by two different sperm. Other than having the same birth date, non-identical twins are genetically no more similar than siblings.

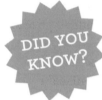

DID YOU KNOW?

Only non-identical twins are hereditary; some women have a genetic predisposition to releasing two eggs. Identical twins, when the fertilised egg splits, are an unusual, unexplained but fortuitous occurrence that does not run in families.

Twin pregnancies are more closely monitored than singletons because of the increased risks to both the mother and her babies. You'll have more appointments and more scans; how many depends on the type of twin pregnancy you're having.

Twin or multiple pregnancies can take three different forms:
- **DCDA** (Dichorionic diamniotic): Each twin has its own placenta and sac. All non-identical twins and a third of identical twins are DCDA. These pregnancies are the most common and the safest. If all is well you'll be scanned every four weeks and there's a good chance you'll go to term and have an uncomplicated twin pregnancy.
- **MCDA** (Monochorionic diamniotic): The twins share a placenta but essentially have their own sac. Two-thirds of identical twins are MCDA. Because the twins are sharing a placenta, these pregnancies are slightly more complicated and it's common to be scanned every two weeks from 16 weeks to keep an eye on things.
- **MCMA** (Monochorionic monoamniotic): The twins share a placenta and a sac. This is very rare; only 1 per cent of identical twins are MCMA. These pregnancies carry higher risks so you will be seen more often and looked after by a specialist team. In fact, current practice is an elective delivery (either induction or caesarean) at 32–33 weeks.

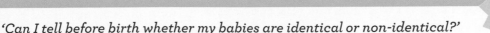

'Can I tell before birth whether my babies are identical or non-identical?'
If your babies are MCDA or MCMA, you will know that they are identical. If they are DCDA, they could be either and the only way to know 100 per cent for certain is to do a DNA test once they're born.

 Tips for twin pregnancies

Carrying twins is more effort so make sure you take extra care to slow down and rest to allow your body to do its job. For the sake of your babies, you should really try to take it easy from 28 weeks, or even earlier depending on the type of pregnancy. We suggest that mothers stop work by about 32 weeks and spend the remainder of their pregnancy resting as much as possible to try to get their babies nice and big when they're born.

Be prepared that many twins arrive earlier than anticipated. Doctors are keen to keep twins in utero as long as possible, and the same gestation of 40 weeks applies to both twins and multiples. However, over half of twins and virtually all triplets are born at or before 37 weeks.

'Will I need to have a caesarean?'
As with all women, the mother's choice of how she would like to give birth plays a large role, and it is certainly possible to have a vaginal birth as long as the medical staff are happy that it's safe. This will depend on the type of twins, their well-being and position, as well as many other factors. Over half of twins and virtually all triplets are born by caesarean. As is the case with all pregnancies, it's important to keep an open mind, and listen to the advice of the team looking after you.

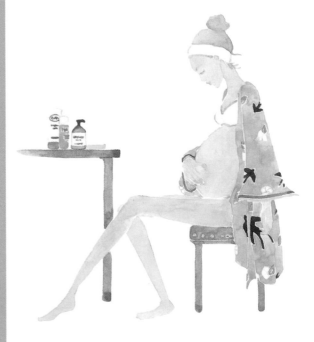

18 Becoming a father:
preparing for fatherhood and supporting your partner

The best thing you can do to prepare for the imminent arrival of your baby is to understand a bit about pregnancy, birth and babies. You may not want to read the whole of this book (and it's not entirely necessary) but it's definitely worth arming yourself with some knowledge. The three 'Becoming a father' chapters cover things from a dad or partner's perspective and, along with the other chapters we've referenced, will provide you with the basics.

Paternal anxiety?

It's not uncommon for fathers to feel a little bit anxious at the news that they will soon become a dad. Try not to worry about the fact that you're nervous; it's entirely normal and remember that you have eight months until the baby is born. Nature has been very clever at making sure parents have time to get used to the idea. Try to talk to friends who are parents; they're often reassuring and also realistic, and they will become a great sounding board and source of advice in the next few years.

Support during the first and second trimesters

Try to be supportive and tolerant in pregnancy. We're sure you're aware of the magnitude of what your partner's body is achieving in these nine months, and it's not uncommon for there to be side effects. The first trimester (3 months) is often really tough – women are surprisingly tired and often really quite sick. By 12 weeks your baby is fully formed and your partner has also grown a placenta, a whole new organ, so it's not surprising that she might feel tired. Encourage her to rest and even have a sleep during the day and to eat little and often. Reassure her that this is all normal and that very soon she'll feel much better. The good news is that the second trimester is when women tend to blossom and feel wonderful.

Support in the third trimester

The last trimester is all about growth. While your baby is getting nice and big, your partner will become increasingly tired, uncomfortable and probably fed up – and this is the time she will really need some support. It is your job (for your baby's sake as well as your partner's) to make sure she slows down:

● Encourage her to stop work earlier than she may think; stopping by 36 weeks is not unreasonable but she really should not be working up until her due date. Even if she doesn't think she will need to stop earlier, she will. Be firm and remind her that by 37 weeks she will be term and the baby may be ready to come.

- Make sure she has a rest and ideally a sleep in the middle of the day. Not only will her sleep be increasingly disturbed at night but it's a good habit to get into – it's something she'll definitely need to be doing once the baby is born.
- Ideally she shouldn't be doing heavy household chores. Vacuuming, emptying the dishwasher or carrying washing upstairs are not going to do her any good at this stage. Remember how much her body is doing just by being pregnant.
- Arrange a relaxing weekend, or even better a week, away. Spend some time enjoying each other's company. Your life is about to change considerably and you should relish the last time you can go away just the two of you without the responsibility of being a parent.

 ## As the birth approaches

- Make sure she's organised and help her get the baby's room ready.
- Work out how the buggy folds and how to put the car seat into the car – this will be your job when the baby comes home from the hospital.
- Try to be excited and positive (even if you're a bit daunted by all the baby paraphernalia).
- Make sure you know where the hospital is and where to park. It won't do any harm to do a practice run or at least work out how to get there.
- Spend some time learning what will happen in labour. You should ideally read pages 116–17, 128–31, 132–33 and 134–37. Don't be afraid to ask any questions but beware of horror stories that your friends might tell you. People love a horror story and these kind of anecdotes tend to become more dramatic the more they are told.
- Try to be positive and look forward to labour – it's going to culminate in the most amazing day of your life!
- Talk about how she would like you to support her in labour. Have frank conversations about where you should be at each stage (i.e. do you want to be at the business end?).
- Keep an open mind and not make too many decisions. Certainly don't hold her to any decisions she may have made in the run-up to labour.

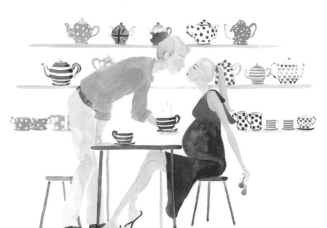

'Don't underestimate the time it takes to put together a buggy and work out how the car seat works. I have a degree in physics and, I swear, this was harder than anything I've had to do professionally ...'
MARK, THE BUMP CLASS

19 You and your baby in the *fourth month* (Weeks 14–17)

Congratulations, you're now entering the second trimester, which is the part of pregnancy most women enjoy the most! Reaching this milestone is exciting. A lot of women don't want to think too much about their pregnancy until after their 12-week scan, so for many the second trimester is when they can finally celebrate their big secret. However good you are at keeping secrets, many might have had a suspicion that you were harbouring exciting news; not drinking, not feeling great and considerable breast growth are all big giveaways.

 Not only does the excitement start but, if you've been feeling rotten in your first trimester, the likelihood is that you'll feel much better in your second. Rather like a hangover finally clearing, morning sickness abating makes pregnant women feel on top of the world. Enjoy this trimester because by the time you reach your third you will start feeling heavy and tired.

 ## How you may be feeling

- If you experienced morning sickness, this is the time most women start to feel better; the nausea subsides and your frequent trips to the loo are less frequent.
- You might have some new strange symptoms though – you could possibly experience nosebleeds, nasal congestion, blocked ears and bleeding gums.
- Towards the end of this month, you might feel butterfly-like flickers in your tummy, which are your fetus' movements.
- Frustratingly you might experience 'baby brain', where even the most efficient, organised and reliable women can suddenly find themselves uncharacteristically forgetful. Frustrating as this is, stressing about it will only make it worse. Have a sense of humour about it, use aids such as lists and electronic reminders to help you get through and, above all, remember that it is temporary!
- As your fetus grows, you will start fitting into fewer of your normal clothes. You will have probably noticed quite significant changes to your body – larger breasts and a thickening of your waist (but it might be some time before you notice an actual bump, and even longer until it's noticeable to others). Maternity jeans with an elasticated waist are usually the first pregnancy buy!

'I was desperate for my bump to appear as soon as possible; I just felt fat. What I really needed was a T-shirt saying 'I'm not fat, I'm pregnant'. But even at 20 weeks there was no discernible bump and I was fed up. It soon appeared though, and ever since I've been trying to get rid of my residual bump. So enjoy being bump-free for as long as it takes – once it appears you'll be hankering after your pre-pregnancy stomach.' MARINA

⭐ Your baby

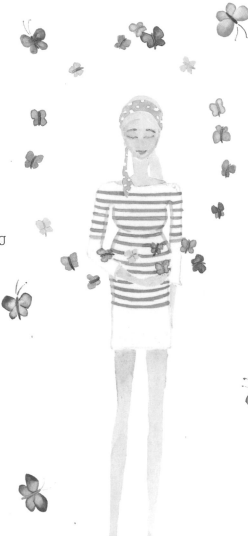

The fetus will start looking more in proportion, with the body now growing faster than the head. If you could see her, you would notice lots of hiccoughing going on, which is actually the fetus practising her breathing movements. This may well continue throughout the pregnancy.

Tiny eyelashes, eyebrows and head hair are developing and her hearing is now pretty good; voices and sounds from the outside world can now be heard! There is a phenomenal amount of growing going on, and by week 17 the fetus weighs around 140 g (5 oz) and is 13 cm (5 inches) long.

20 Antenatal *classes*

It's a good idea to start researching antenatal classes soon, as the good ones tend to get booked up early. Ask friends who live close by to recommend a good class.

We might be biased (!) but a good antenatal class is essential. However much you think you know, a really good class will prepare you for coping with the end of your pregnancy, labour and the first few months as a mother. Make sure the one you choose offers advice from professionals. You should be getting a rounded view of what birth is like in all eventualities and don't let anyone make you feel like you have somehow failed if you don't want to or can't do everything 'naturally'. Too many classes simply focus on natural birth because that is all the girls want to hear about. As a first-time mother in the UK you have a 35 per cent chance of your birth being assisted in some way, so it is best to be prepared.

'I was really reluctant to do an antenatal class; I didn't really have the time and felt I had better things to spend money on. But a good friend persuaded me and, honestly, it was the best decision of my pregnancy. Having been a bit of a reluctant mother-to-be, I spent a lot of my pregnancy annoyed at all the things I couldn't do. Spending one morning a week with 10 pregnant women learning about what my body was doing and how to prepare made me, for the first time, really excited about becoming a mother. And, even better, the girls I met shared the pivotal experience of becoming a mother with me – we became great friends and an invaluable support network.' MARINA

Dealing with 'helpful' advice

As you become visibly pregnant, you will start to attract advice, tips and judgement from others. This is often conflicting, inaccurate and unwelcome. People love to tell a good horror story – one that might have been based on truth but that has invariably lost nothing in the telling. It's just not what you need to be hearing. Try to find one person that you take advice from – it might be your antenatal teacher, a good friend or your doctor – and ignore everything else.

21 Baby *movements*

Feeling that first little kick is something most mothers never forget. It is a very real reminder that there is a little person growing inside you, and all those early pregnancy symptoms suddenly seem worth it!

The stage at which you first feel your baby's movements vary from woman to woman and it will depend on various factors like how active your baby is, how big she is and how big you are. However, most first movements are felt at around 17 weeks. Your baby's movements will change as she grows.

- **First movements** (around 17 weeks): Most mothers describe the first movements as like butterflies (or wind), and initially it can be hard to know if they really were movements at all. Very quickly, however, they develop a pattern and a familiarity that you will get to know and find very comforting.

- **Mid pregnancy:** As your baby gets stronger and still has room to move about she will start giving you little punches, which can actually be quite uncomfortable, particularly if they are in the ribs or into a full bladder! This is the stage where you can often begin to see baby movements through the tummy, and some parents have even reported seeing tiny hand- or footprints through the skin!

- **Late pregnancy:** Towards the end of the pregnancy there is not much space left for your baby to move around, and the movements will usually feel more sweeping. At this stage, during an active time for your baby, it is not uncommon to lie down and be able to see your tummy moving in all sorts of directions as your baby flexes her muscles.

Hiccoughs

Babies are prone to hiccoughs while they are developing – this actually plays an important part in their lung development and practising for when they will take their first breaths. That said, please don't lose sleep if you never feel your baby hiccoughing. She will be doing it without you feeling it. Your baby hiccoughing is an unusual sensation of regular movements and is sometimes confused by pregnant women to be muscle spasms. Lots of babies choose night-time to start hiccoughing – another thing to keep you up at night!

Tracking your baby's movements

Your baby's movements change throughout your pregnancy but there will be a pattern that your recognise.

> *'I commonly see pregnant women who are worried about their baby's movements and this is understandable. It is the only way we as mothers can be reassured that our baby is alive and well. If more time than usual goes by without a movement it can be very nerve-racking. Often drinking a cold or fizzy drink or eating something sugary will encourage a bit of reassuring fetal movement, but if you are concerned get checked out. Most GPs and all midwives and obstetricians have Doppler ultrasound machines to detect the baby's heart rate and will advise you as to whether there is any cause for concern.'* CHIARA

Safety note

If your baby's pattern of movement changes suddenly, or particularly slows down, you should have a check-up.

The most important thing is to trust your instinct, particularly as you get further along in the pregnancy. No one will ever berate you for coming in 'unnecessarily'.

If you are not sure (and you are more than 28 weeks pregnant), the advice is to lie down on your left side for 2 hours and count the separate movements. If there are less than 10 movements, you should have a check-up.

Q&A

'Should I buy my own Doppler machine to reassure myself?'
This is a difficult one and it very much depends on your personality and the circumstances. It is not always easy to find the baby's heartbeat using an ultrasound, and I have come across many panicked mothers who have bought a machine and then rushed to see me in a panic when they haven't found the heartbeat, which was there all along. It is also easy to start becoming obsessed with the machine and worrying when the heartrate rises or falls, not really knowing how to interpret it, or even getting it confused with your own heartbeat. That said, in some circumstances it can be useful, so discuss it with the medical professional looking after you.

22 Dressing your *bump*

At some point in the second trimester your eagerly awaited bump will emerge. It's impossible for us to give you the week in which that will occur – it's amazing how it differs not only between women but also between pregnancies. For some a bump will start to appear shortly after 12 weeks but for many it won't really be visible until after 20 weeks.

Then begins the difficulty of dressing your bump. A lot of women find their shape changes before a bump appears, and it's not uncommon to need new jeans before 12 weeks. One way of clinging on to your favourite pair for slightly longer is to invest in an 'extender', which essentially expands the waist of your jeans. For some girls, their whole body will have become larger, due to hormonal changes and increased water retention, and it will be the thighs that don't fit. If you have had a small waist you'll probably notice your body change faster than those who have skinny legs and less of a waist. In the early stages, rather than buying a whole lot of pregnancy clothes, it will be more a case of editing your wardrobe to fit your slightly altered shape.

As you progress into your second trimester, you will have to start investing in maternity clothes. Thankfully there is a far bigger choice of clothes for pregnant women now than ten years ago. A good pair of maternity jeans is an essential, and many of you will love how comfy they are. They will have a stretchy waistband – some are thin and go under your bump but others cover your bump entirely. Be wary of these in the summer, as covering your whole bump can get hot.

You'll also need to invest in some pregnancy tops – simple T-shirts and vest tops work well as you can then put your favourite cardigans or tops over them. A lot of girls find wearing a tight top with a cardigan emphasises their bump, making them look pregnant rather than just fat.

Do remember that you don't just need to wear pregnancy clothes. Loose-fitting dresses worn with a belt on your new waistline – just above your bump – is a good way of emphasising your pregnancy.

Belts with a little stretch work well for this or you could just use a simple ribbon – a good haberdasher's will always have a selection to brighten outfits. Do try on maxi dresses – the naturally higher waistline is often really flattering for pregnant women, and again these don't need to be specifically maternity.

There comes a time when you want to spoil yourself and buy a lovely piece of clothing. Rather than buying something that you will only be able to wear in your pregnancy, think instead of buying a good jacket or cardigan that you can wear open in pregnancy and continue to wear after your baby is born.

Most women's breasts grow significantly the moment they conceive and continue to do so throughout their pregnancy. It's really important to wear a well-fitting bra. Not only will your breasts become important feeding vessels in a matter of months but a good bra will make you look infinitely slimmer. You can buy bra extenders that make them bigger around the rib cage but do make sure your bra fits around the breasts. It's fine to continue to wear underwired bras in pregnancy as long as they fit really well. If in doubt, get measured. There's no need to buy expensive underwear; you'll only wear it for a short period of time (your breasts might well continue to grow in your pregnancy). Instead you can save up for some nice post-pregnancy lingerie.

 Your work wardrobe

- Try to make your old clothes last as long as possible using waist expanders, elastic bands or even safety pins.
- When you absolutely need to invest in new items, try getting five or six pieces in the same or complementary colours that you can mix and match.
- Accessories are key. Not only will they make a boring outfit appear glamorous but by changing your accessories you'll be able to get away with fewer outfits. Think about belts, shoes, scarves, bags and jewellery. Don't be afraid to go bold!
- If you are used to wearing high heels at work you may have to rethink this. See the box opposite for tips on pregnancy footwear.

'*What shoes should I wear in pregnancy?*'

Because of the hormonal changes that take place from right at the beginning of your pregnancy, you are more prone to injury and therefore you do need to think carefully about what shoes you are wearing. In an ideal world, all pregnant women would immediately ditch the high heels and instead stick to sensible shoes that support your feet. But life isn't always about doing the most sensible thing; sometimes you just need that bit of extra glamour, height or indulgence in pregnancy so we're not going to tell you just to wear Velcro sandals with a supportive heel. Instead, bear the following in mind:

- If you want to wear heels regularly, for example at work, invest in a lower heel.
- Try to ensure heels are as supportive as possible – instead of a stiletto with a strappy back, choose a platform with a thicker heel or a wedge.
- When wearing heels, have a back-up pair of shoes with you for when you can't stand them any more. Flimsy ballerinas are not the ideal shoe in pregnancy as they don't provide a lot of support, but you probably won't be able to fit your Birkenstocks into your clutch bag, so ballerinas are better than nothing.
- Try not to walk very far in heels and sit down as much as you can.
- If you do need to walk, it's the time to wear sensible shoes. Put on your trainers and change if necessary when you get wherever you're going.

 Summer clothes

- Maxi dresses
- Kaftans
- Leggings worn under a tunic
- Bigger bikinis or, if you can't face exposing your belly, a tankini or swimsuit designed for pregnancy
- Hat – this is essential as your skin is more sensitive to the sun in pregnancy
- Maternity shorts – mercifully cool for the perpetually hot pregnant woman
- Accessories: use sandals, bags, belts/ribbons, scarves and sunglasses to glam up an otherwise dull pregnancy outfit

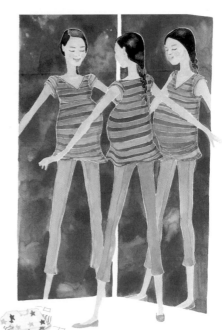

 Winter clothes

- Jeans
- Boots that are easy to get into
- Pregnancy vest tops and good cardigans

- Coat: don't specifically buy a pregnancy coat but choose something with a shape that will naturally accommodate your bump. There are plenty around and this will last you after your pregnancy
- Tights (pregnancy tights can have a habit of falling down so you might want to just go for a size up – they're very stretchy after all!)
- Accessories: use hats, jewellery and belts

⭐ Dressing your bump for a smart event

- **Don't limit yourself to the pregnancy ranges:** Rather than buying something specifically for pregnancy that you will never wear again, try to look for something which will embrace your bump. Not only is the choice in non-maternity clothes much bigger but chances are you'll be able to wear it again, justifying the price. Look out for dresses with empire lines or something with a belt that you can adjust.
- **Accessorise!** Buy something simple and spend money on the accessories. Treat yourself to a killer necklace that will become a focal point.
- **Divert attention to your assets.** For most women their hair while pregnant is thick, shiny and looks amazing. Spoil yourself with a blow-dry and make your lustrous locks the focus of your look.
- **Be realistic about heels:** If possible stick to flats, but if you really must wear heels, see the box on page 63 for advice.

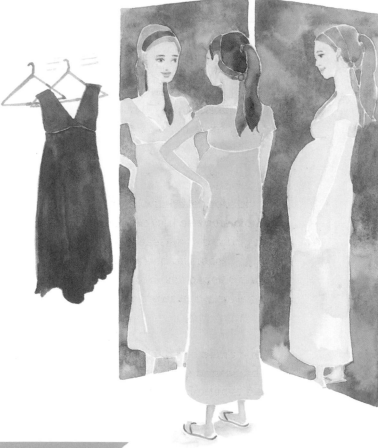

23 Working while you're pregnant

Sharing pregnancy news with workplaces differs dramatically. Some workplaces are family-friendly and have huge experience in dealing with pregnancy within the workforce. For others, pregnancy seems to be a whispered faux pas – something that is unofficially frowned upon. While it's not often a good idea to announce your exciting news before you've reached the critical 12-week mark, with the debilitating symptoms so common in the first trimester, it's often hard to hide the fact that you are pregnant.

You must inform your employer of your pregnancy at least 15 weeks before your due date. In most uncomplicated pregnancies, that means 15 weeks before 40 weeks, so by the start of your twenty-fifth week of pregnancy. However, because you're entitled to time off for antenatal appointments, you might want to tell your workplace sooner.

 ## Announcing your pregnancy at work

When considering when to break the news, do bear a few things in mind:

- Make sure it's your boss who knows first. Schedule a meeting with your boss and confirm your announcement in writing.
- It's important that they hear the news from you, rather than unofficially on the office grapevine or because your usually flat tummy has turned into an unmistakeable pregnancy bump. The law prevents your employer making potentially negative decisions about your job as a result of your pregnancy, but if your employer knows or suspects before your official announcement, you're not so well protected.
- Consider the timing of your announcement. If it comes just after you've completed a successful project, you can emphasise that your pregnancy will not affect your work. Similarly, try to get any reviews out of the way so that you're judged on your past work, rather than any concerns about your future abilities.
- If your job is very physical or involves exposure to potentially harmful products, you should tell your employer much sooner. Similarly if you're really feeling atrocious in the first trimester, it might be best to share the good news with them earlier so that they can support and understand you. It's worth asking for discretion until you reach 12 weeks.
- Know your rights; make sure you do some research and find out what you are legally entitled to and what your company policy is. If you can speak to an employee who has experienced pregnancy in your company, as long as you can trust them to be utterly discreet, it might be useful to pick their brains about how your employer dealt with and reacted to their pregnancy.

● Start making a plan. At some point you will need to agree when you will take your maternity leave. We see a lot of Bump Class girls take the decision in their second trimester (when they are feeling great) to continue to work right up until their due date. What they haven't anticipated is how tired they will start to feel after around week 34. If at all possible, do consider taking maternity leave from 34–36 weeks. Not only will it do both you and the baby good to rest, but you've also got a lot to organise before your baby arrives. Don't forget, you're actually at term from 37 weeks, and even though first babies are more likely to be late, many do arrive before the much-anticipated 40 weeks.

 Your maternity leave

A lot of employers will ask you to tell them when you intend to go back to work. Before you've had your baby, know that it's healthy and are familiar with the rigours and sleeplessness of motherhood, it's impossible to know what is realistic. Luckily the government protects mothers from having to make this decision too early. Legally your employer has to assume a mother will take the full allowed 52 weeks unless they are told otherwise. If you're planning to go back to work before then, you need to give your employer at least eight weeks' notice. Please do take advantage of this legislation; it's in place because it's impossible for a mother to make this decision before she's had her baby.

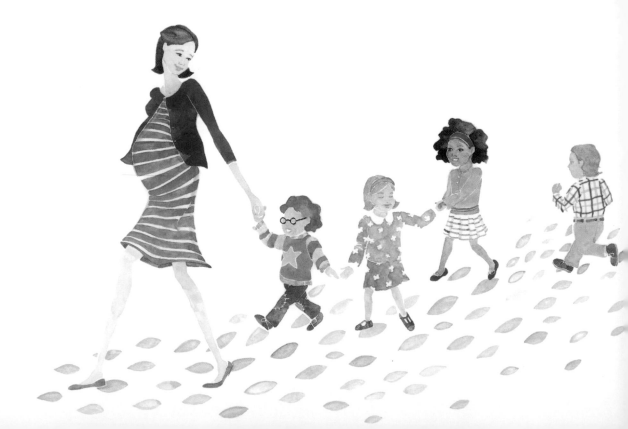

24 When to see *your doctor*

How do you know if a new pregnancy symptom is something to worry about or just part of being pregnant? Our advice is always to mention any symptom you are concerned about at your next doctor or midwife appointment. If that is a while away and you have concerns, your doctor or midwife will be very happy to see you.

On the next few pages are a few symptoms, which, if you experience, you should always report to your doctor or midwife as soon as possible. They don't always mean that there is something wrong but medical staff will need to exclude any serious problems that could be causing them.

It's never good to worry excessively in pregnancy; stress isn't any good for you or your baby. So, while we don't want to scare you, it is best to be aware of the things you should immediately report to your doctor.

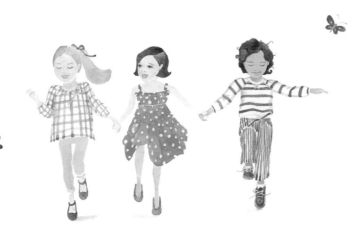

What	Why
Any form of vaginal bleeding at any stage of the pregnancy	There are lots of reasons for this depending on the stage of your pregnancy, from miscarriage to a low-lying placenta or small change in the cervix. In many cases you and your baby will be fine but it's not normal and should always be checked out
Anything that could be your waters breaking (bear in mind this may not be a big gush – see page 128)	Ideally we don't want your waters to break until the baby is ready to be delivered, so if it looks like this is happening early, see someone straight away
Profuse or smelly vaginal discharge	This could be a sign of a vaginal infection, which can usually be easily treated
Cramping abdominal pain, particularly if it's getting worse or coming regularly	The worry is that these could be contractions coming early
Worsening headache, especially if you're also experiencing any upper abdominal pain or swelling of face, hands and feet, or visual symptoms, e.g. blurred vision or flashing lights	These can be signs of pre-eclampsia
General swelling. Although it's common for women to have to take off their rings and put up with swollen ankles in the third trimester, if it happens suddenly and you feel unwell make sure you see someone. Severe itching, particularly on your palms and soles	We worry that these could be signs of pre-eclampsia. There are many causes of itching in pregnancy, ranging from eczema to obstetric cholestasis, a potentially serious liver disorder which would need to be treated in hospital. Fifteen per cent of women suffer itching in pregnancy, and in the majority this is not serious, but it's worth getting it checked if it's particularly severe

What	Why
Not feeling your baby move for a prolonged period. As you get bigger you will learn the pattern of your baby's movements and will recognise if these change. It is very difficult to generalise but if you notice a significant change in this pattern, particularly if the movements seem to be fewer than normal, you should contact your hospital. Your mother's instinct is very strong; trust it. (See page 60 for more on this.)	The reasons for this are wide-ranging and could simply be that as the baby grows there is less space for her to move around or she's just having a sleepy day. But sometimes it can also be an indication that something is seriously wrong which could potentially lead to stillbirth. For this reason, if you have any concerns you should always get checked out
If you are unwell with a fever (around 37°C/98.6°F is normal; 38°C/100.4°F and above is a fever)	Fever is an indication that there is an infection which needs to be diagnosed and treated promptly
If you suddenly develop a swollen leg on one side	You're at increased risk of blood clots in pregnancy. If a clot gets lodged in the leg, it can produce these symptoms, which, although rare, are potentially very dangerous
If you become suddenly short of breath or have chest pain	These could be symptoms of a blood clot in the lung, which, although rare, is a risk for pregnant women
If you just don't feel quite right	Please remember that this is not an exhaustive list. The key is to contact your healthcare provider if you have any concerns, even if you can't put your finger on it. If you call up a hospital, you will not be waking anyone up and if they check you over and all is fine, no one will accuse you of wasting their time

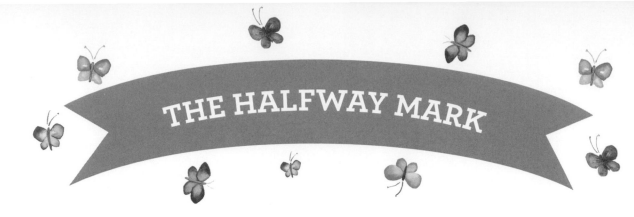

THE HALFWAY MARK

25 You and your baby in the *fifth month* (Weeks 18–21)

 How you may be feeling

- You are likely to be noticeably bigger, with often some achiness in the lower abdomen or ribs where your ligaments are beginning to stretch to accommodate your growing fetus.
- Your appetite might well have increased.
- You may find that your libido is back, having dropped off a bit in the last few months. However, many women also find that they have no sex drive at all at this stage. Remember that both are normal in pregnancy and it is important to discuss it with your partner. (See page 80 for more on sex and pregnancy.)
- You may start to experience the delights of varicose veins or haemorrhoids – if these start causing a problem speak to your GP.
- Stretch marks might appear as your fetus' growth accelerates. Whether or not you get these is largely to do with your genes (see page 78). Unfortunately they will not disappear after the delivery of the baby but they will fade.
- You may also be developing an 'outie', as your pregnancy pushes your tummy button out. This will go back in once the baby is born, although it may not quite return to its pre-pregnancy look.
- Between weeks 19 and 21 you will have your second and final routine scan, the 20-week scan (see page 72).

Your baby

There is likely to be a lot more activity this month, and it is when most women start feeling movements for the first time. As the brain is developing, the fetus is becoming more coordinated and is now capable of various gymnastic moves, including somersaults. She will also be practising movements such as punching, kicking, rolling, twisting, grasping, sucking and swallowing, as well as beginning to make and practise different facial expressions! She will begin to have well-defined periods of wakefulness and sleep, which, if you are lucky, might fit in with yours!

Your fetus will develop 'lanugo' (a fine downy hair that covers her) at around five months. This hair acts as an 'anchor' for the 'vernix' (a thick white greasy substance that protects the baby in the womb and keeps it warm). The lanugo usually begins to fall out at around month eight or nine, but some babies are born with it and it subsequently falls out in the first few weeks.

The genitals are now well developed, although a boy's testicles will not have descended into the scrotum yet. A girl will have a fully developed uterus by now and there will be a lifetime's supply of eggs in her ovaries (over 3 million). By the end of month five the fetus now weighs about 360 g (13 oz) and is about 26 cm (10 in) long.

26 The 20-week scan (anomaly scan)

⭐ **What they're checking for**

For most women the 12-week scan is the green light to celebrate and get excited about being pregnant. But eight weeks later you have another ultrasound scan that looks closely at how the fetus and all her organs are developing. Rather than just a quick look to see if all is well or simply to tell you the sex of your fetus, at the 20-week scan the sonographer will spend a lot of time looking at your fetus' various organs to check that they are developing as they should.

What will be checked
- Head and brain
- Heart – its chambers, valves and blood vessels
- Abdominal contents, particularly kidneys and stomach
- Spine
- Facial features
- Hands and feet
- Placenta, umbilical cord and amniotic fluid
- Genitals – this is usually the time they can let you know whether you're having a boy or a girl.

Unfortunately it's at this scan that abnormalities are sometimes found. Most irregular findings are minor and may require re-scanning or surgery but will not necessarily affect the outcome of your pregnancy. In some cases the abnormalities are potentially life-threatening. This is devastating for parents, but the teams specially trained to support couples at this time offer excellent care.

Do remember that these cases are very rare indeed. In the UK we're so lucky to be at the cutting edge of science, and every precaution is taken to ensure that our babies arrive in our arms fit and healthy. For most mothers, the 20-week scan is an amazing window into their uterus, where they can see their perfect little baby growing beautifully. So enjoy it and be prepared to get emotional.

A note on ultrasounds

Ultrasound scans have been used in pregnancy since the mid 1950s and have no known side effects for mother or baby. They're a really good way of having a non-invasive yet detailed look inside the uterus at the developing fetus.

It is important to remember that, although the scans are very good, they do not always detect every abnormality. A normal scan, although very reassuring, does not give a 100 per cent clean bill of health. For example, of the 1 per cent of babies born with a heart abnormality, only about half of these are picked up in the scan – the rest are picked up at birth or later. The scans only look at the structure of the organs but can't give us much information about their function; this can be more carefully assessed after the baby is born.

Q&A

'I was told my placenta is "low lying" on my 12-week scan. Will it still be low at my 20-week scan and what does that mean for my birth and my baby?'
Ideally we want the placenta to be high up in the uterus. Most placentas that are low at 12 weeks have moved up by 20 weeks. However, if it hasn't, don't panic; there is a good chance that it still will and a further scan will be organised at about 34 weeks to see if it has moved up. If you are one of the 50 per cent whose placentas have not moved by the time your baby is due, you will be advised to have a caesarean.

N.B If the placenta is low and partially or totally covering the cervix it is called 'placenta praevia'. This happens in about 0.5 per cent of women. If this is the case the main risk is painless vaginal bleeding late in pregnancy. You should see a doctor immediately if this happens. If there is no bleeding there is no risk to the baby or to you, although you will be advised to have a caesarean.

'I want to know the sex of the baby but my husband doesn't. What do we do?'
This was the dilemma one of our Bump Class girls faced. She decorated the nursery in neutral colours and had a special drawer with any gender-specific baby items that her husband was told to stay away from. Remarkably restrained, he didn't find out that his baby was a boy until his birth!

27 You and your baby in the *sixth month* (Weeks 22–26)

The big milestone this month is reaching 24 weeks, when your baby is for the first time considered by the medical world as 'viable'. This means that, if she were to be born, she would have a chance of surviving outside the womb. Although no one would choose for their baby to be born this early on, it's a landmark stage of your pregnancy.

 How you may be feeling

- Many women notice **skin changes** this month – see page 76 for more on the kind of changes you might experience.
- **Leg cramps** at night can become more debilitating as your pregnancy progresses. You can relieve these by doing stretches and wearing support stockings.
- You may have an **itchy tummy**; as the skin across your bump becomes more taught it becomes more dry, often resulting in annoyingly itchy skin. Try not to scratch. Massaging your abdomen with oil or calamine lotion can help. If you have itching all over your body you should see your doctor.
- By the end of this month your uterus is about the size of a football and you will be noticeably **heavier** and **more cumbersome**.
- You might feel **breathless**; as your uterus grows, it presses up against your diaphragm, leaving less room for your lungs to expand.
- You may notice that you have become **clumsier**, dropping things or tripping over more often. You can blame this on your hormones, which are causing your joints to loosen and your hands to swell. Don't worry, your pre-pregnancy dexterity will return again, we promise!

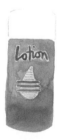

THE BUMP CLASS

Your baby

- Your baby's eyes can open and close now and she will be able to tell the difference between light and dark. If you shine a torch onto your bump and move it, she may turn her head to follow it or may even use her hands to shield her eyes from the light.
- She will continue to be increasingly mobile and dexterous, opening and closing her fist and curling her toes. She may regularly interlock her fingers or grasp hold of the umbilical cord as it floats past. You may now start to feel her hiccoughs. They are usually felt as regular intermittent spasms.
- Your baby's vocal cords are now fully functional, although she won't make her first sound until she is born.
- The hair on her head is still white as no pigment has been deposited yet, and her skin is still very thin and translucent as there is not yet any fat underneath it.
- At 26 weeks your baby will weigh around 760 g (27 oz) and be about 35 cm (14 inches) from head to toe.

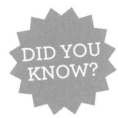

DID YOU KNOW?

Until 24 weeks fetal length is generally measured from crown (head) to rump (bottom). After 24 weeks the baby is more stretched out, so length is measured from head to heel.

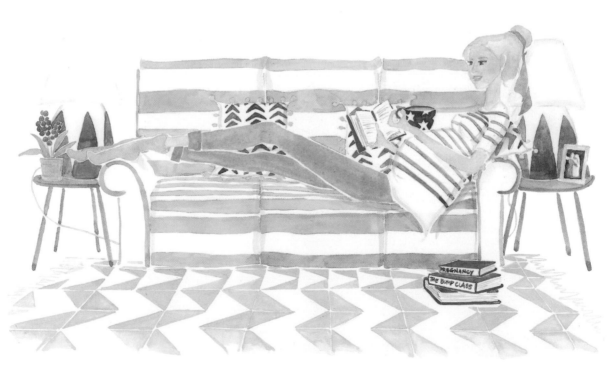

28 Beauty in *pregnancy*

'Girl babies "steal" their mother's beauty' is a myth we often hear. For the lucky women, pregnancy brings with it an ethereal glow which lasts throughout their pregnancy, and for others it is quite the opposite. There is no evidence to suggest that a mother's physical appearance has any bearing on the sex of her child but one thing we can tell you is that wincing every time you catch a glimpse of yourself in the mirror is not fun.

Hormonal changes in pregnancy affect your skin and hair profoundly. Here are some of the changes you might notice.

 ## Hair

Most girls' hair in pregnancy is thick, bouncy and shiny, but for some unlucky others, who may have had amazing hair beforehand, it turns limp and frizzy. However, your hair is likely to go back to normal at some point after childbirth.

Very little research has been done into the safety of using hair chemicals in pregnancy. Although some are probably safe to use, others could contain chemicals that could be absorbed through the scalp and potentially cause harm. For this reason we'd advise avoiding any chemical hair treatments during pregnancy, particularly in the first trimester. If going without isn't an option, highlights and natural dyes are generally considered safe. Do make sure though that you're sitting in a well-ventilated area and not breathing in too many fumes.

 ## Skin

The most common skin change in pregnancy is discolouration. Freckles and moles often get darker, as does the nipple area. Some women experience large areas of skin discolouration – either from dark to light in dark-skinned women or light to dark in light-skinned women. This can occur on the face, when it's called 'cholasma' or 'the mask of pregnancy'. You may also have noticed a dark line appear between your belly button and your pubic bone. This is known as a 'linea negra', and it's actually the darkening of a usually invisible line, the 'linea alba'. These skin changes are

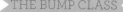
THE BUMP CLASS

all caused by your raging hormones so there's not a lot that can be done about them; however, your skin should return to normal in the first six months after your pregnancy.

Exposure to the sun often exacerbates any skin changes you might be experiencing, so make sure you wear sunscreen the whole time and try to keep out of the sun as much as possible.

'One of the first signs I'm pregnant is a breakout of spots, which tends to stay with me until the end of my pregnancy. These are large, red, unsightly blights on my face and do nothing for my self-esteem. Reluctant to use any medication I experimented with various natural things and my solution was a tea tree oil stick for spots, which tended to zap them brilliantly.' OLIVIA, BUMP CLASS

Skincare products and pregnancy

As your skin is more sensitive in pregnancy, it's worth exercising a degree of caution with the products that you use. Do make sure that your doctor has okayed any medicated products you're using. Where day-to-day skincare products are concerned, we recommend that you don't need to stop using something unless it becomes problematic. If you're finding that you're suddenly reacting to creams you used to be fine with, steer towards unscented products where possible.

 ## Eczema

Eczema sufferers often find that their eczema flares up during their pregnancy, partly due to the pregnancy and partly because they are trying to avoid using their medicated creams, which they are told to avoid in pregnancy. If you find your eczema is really flaring up again, please talk to your doctor, who will probably advise a steroid cream. This is another situation where the risk of harm to your baby from the steroid cream (very small) is probably outweighed by the risk to your baby from you being exhausted from not sleeping and sore from scratching as well as the risk of infection.

 ## Varicose veins

Varicose veins are another treat that may spring up in pregnancy. If you are suffering you should keep off your legs as much as possible and wear support stockings (as hideous as they are). The likelihood is that they will massively improve after the baby is born, but if they don't there are lots of other treatment options once you are no longer pregnant.

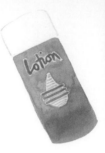

Less commonly talked about but also a possibility are vulval varicose veins, which can also be very uncomfortable. They generally feel like an aching discomfort in the perineal area, particularly when standing up. Avoiding standing for long periods and wearing supportive underwear can help. Thankfully, this does improve after your baby has been born.

 ## Stretch marks

For many, the prospect of getting stretch marks in pregnancy is worse than the idea of cellulite. Unfortunately 90 per cent of us do develop stretch marks. While they may be red, angry and itchy during pregnancy, after birth they tend to subside and after a few months are subtle and silvery in their appearance. Whether or not you get stretch marks is largely determined by genetics, although there is some evidence to suggest that stretch marks are caused by the rapid stretching of skin and therefore those who combine a healthy diet (not putting on too much weight) with exercise (keeping your muscles strong) are less prone to them.

Moisturising every day will not prevent stretch marks but there's certainly no harm in doing so; in fact, as your bump grows, regular moisturising will prevent itchiness and allow you to spend time enjoying your growing bump. There are lots of expensive oils on the market but there is little good evidence to suggest these are any more beneficial than very simple, inexpensive products.

If, after your pregnancy, you're really unhappy about your stretch marks, do talk to your doctor as there are some things that can be done with laser therapy to reduce their appearance.

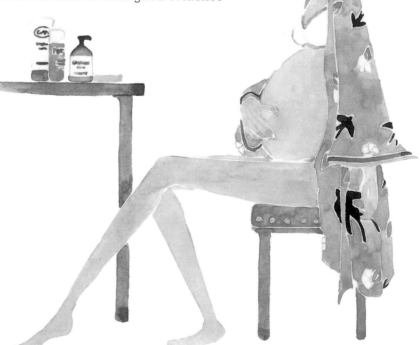

29 Your emotional side *during pregnancy*

Nearly all pregnant women are floored by their heightened emotions. Often this is one of the first symptoms and it can be confusing before you even know you're pregnant. It's definitely something to warn your partner about but, don't worry, you have not turned into a fragile, weeping woman forever (although be prepared, being a mother will make you always vulnerable to emotional stories involving innocent children).

'For me, the first sign of pregnancy, was my tears at a ... wait for it ... health insurance advert! Thereafter romcoms were off limits, and when it came to sick children, I couldn't even hear a story.' MARINA

Grumpiness is also common, especially as your pregnancy progresses. It's not a huge surprise when you think about it as day-to-day life is becoming considerably harder. You're fat, bloated, tired, constantly on the loo and, when you're not, you don't have enough energy to have any fun. Understanding that you need to slow down will ease the grumpiness but you should also make sure that those around you understand that it's largely caused by your hormones. Rather than berate you, make sure they reassure you and encourage you to slow down if necessary.

'In the latter stages of my first pregnancy, unable to find a parking space at the supermarket, I spotted a "mother and baby" slot, perfect for manoeuvring my bump out of the car. As I marched into the shop, I was stopped by a parking attendant who cautiously asked, "Excuse me, madam, do you have a child with you?" I turned around and glared at him. "I think it should be perfectly obvious that my child is in my uterus." The jaw of this overzealous parking warden hit the floor as I strode off, delighted with my interpretation of the rules, even if my manners may have temporarily deserted me.' MARINA

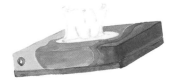

30 Sex and *pregnancy*

Delighted mothers often rave about their increased sex drives and heightened sexual pleasure in pregnancy, but this is not the case for all, and it often changes during pregnancy. For many women, who are plagued by incessant nausea and drop-dead tiredness in the first trimester, sex is not something high on their agenda when they finally get into bed. Often when the early pregnancy symptoms subside, in the second trimester, you can fully enjoy the increased sensitivity that the hormonal changes in pregnancy bring. Unfortunately in the third trimester the returning fatigue, plus your increasing bulk, often mean that sex is not quite as regular as it might have been.

Ultimately, sex is different for different couples – largely because, even when you're not pregnant, sex varies in terms of frequency and enjoyment. Generally what's good for the mother is good for the baby, so try to enjoy it but don't force it, and be mindful that your appetite and enjoyment may well wax and wane as your pregnancy progresses.

Unless your doctor has told you otherwise, sex is not only completely safe for you and your baby throughout pregnancy but also really good for all concerned. The baby has no awareness of what is happening and orgasm, however mind-blowing, should not stimulate early labour. Best of all, it's possibly the most enjoyable and fun form of exercise, so feel free to indulge, certainly while you can!

'After our third Bump Class we all went and had a coffee together and we started talking about how we were all finding sex now that we were pregnant. It was really interesting how much we all fluctuated – some girls loved it and were far more active than before and a couple of others really hated having sex. It was a combination of exhaustion, lack of confidence about their changing bodies and, of course, the hormones. We'd talked about how your sex life can change hugely in The Bump Class and what we'd learnt is that everyone is different, but the key is to talk about it with our partners. After our children were born, we all returned to having sex at different times and for each of us it returned to normal, in spite of our worries.' ANONYMOUS (FOR THE SAKE OF THE OTHERS ...)

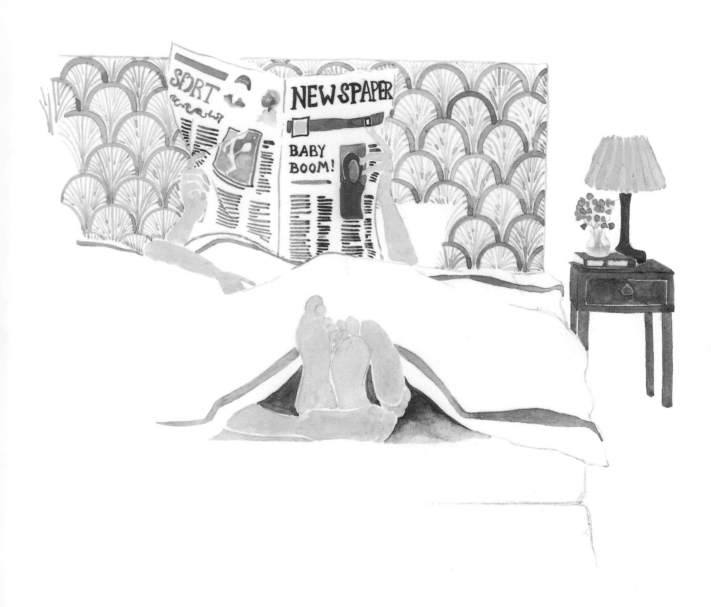

31 You and your baby in the *seventh month* (Weeks 27–30)

You've finally reached your third trimester; this trimester is all about your baby getting nice and big – ready for the outside world. And as a result you will be getting big too! A large healthy baby is what every mother wants, so give your body to chance to make this happen. It's time to start slowing down.

 ## How you may be feeling

- Your pregnancy glow might start to fade.
- You might have the occasional hardening of your stomach; these are Braxton Hicks contractions – your body's way of practising for birth. Some women barely notice them, and for others they are more uncomfortable and can make them think labour has arrived early.
- You are likely to feel increasingly tired, especially if you're having difficulty sleeping; as you get bigger you'll be more uncomfortable. Try to have naps during the day if possible.
- You may be increasingly short of breath.
- Swelling, particularly of hands, feet and legs, is common. Remember to get those rings off your fingers while you can!
- Bloating is also very common in pregnancy. Not only is the growing baby compressing all your abdominal organs but your digestive system is slowing down. These combined mean that food takes longer to travel through the stomach and intestines, often causing symptoms of bloating, tummy ache and, more likely than not, constipation.
- Heartburn is another joy of pregnancy. The valve at the top of your stomach becomes less effective in pregnancy and allows the stomach acid to regurgitate back up, causing a very uncomfortable burning sensation at the front of the chest, particularly when lying flat. Try propping yourself up in bed, eating little and often and drinking milk before meals. If this is not helping speak to your doctor about using an antacid or other treatment.

'Little things may really irritate you. Lying in bed one morning, I heard my husband going for a pee. It seemed to last about five minutes and all I could think was, "That is SO unfair." I was actually jealous of my husband's bladder capacity.' MARINA

Nutrition in your third trimester

During your final trimester it is important to eat and drink plenty of calcium, which is being used to mature and harden your baby's skeleton. Calcium-rich foods include milk, cheese, yogurt, sardines and green vegetables, as well as fortified foods such as cereals, breads and orange juice.

 ## Antenatal check-ups

Your check-up this month will involve the usual blood-pressure check and urine test as well as monitoring the baby's size, position and heart rate. In the third trimester the doctors and midwives will be even more interested in your blood pressure and urine as they can give clues as to whether or not you might be developing pre-eclampsia (see page 38).

The check-up this month will also include a glucose tolerance test to screen for gestational diabetes, a type of diabetes women can get when they are pregnant. Don't worry if you have it, it goes away once you have given birth and the doctors take extra special care of you during your pregnancy and labour. During this check-up, you may also be offered a blood test for anaemia, and if your blood type is rhesus negative you may be offered an anti D injection (see page 49), although the timing of this differs slightly from area to area.

 ## Your baby

At seven months your baby is almost fully developed. If she were born now she would have a good chance of survival.

Your baby will still be very active at this stage, and you will feel lots of strong movements. Every baby's movement pattern is different and there is no set number of movements to feel each day.

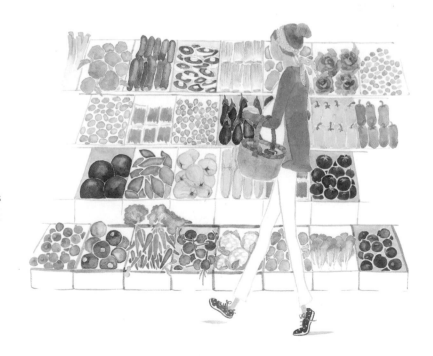

What is important is what is normal for your baby, and any significant change should be reported to your doctor or midwife (see page 60 for further advice on this).

Your baby's brain is developing, and research suggests that from this stage babies begin to develop a primitive form of memory. Your baby can open and close her eyes (and flutter her eyelashes) and is beginning to see. She may be looking at her hands, feet or floating umbilical cord! She has developed a sucking reflex and may even have found her thumb to suck in the womb.

Her hearing is good and the sounds she will be used to are of your heartbeat and breathing, tummy gurgles and swishing water, as well as noises from the outside world. She can now differentiate voices and will be able to recognise them after birth. Some mothers find their babies respond with excited kicks when certain music is played.

By 30 weeks, your baby will weigh about 1.3 kg (3 lb), and when stretched from head to toe may measure up to 41 cm (16 inches) long.

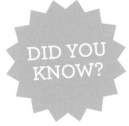

DID YOU KNOW?

By the seventh month your baby's taste buds are developed so she can taste the food you eat through the amniotic fluid she is drinking!

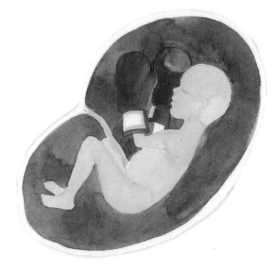

32 Sleeping *in pregnancy*

Considering how important sleep is in pregnancy, it feels really unfair that a lot of women have trouble sleeping at some point during their pregnancy. There are some that say that it's nature's way of preparing you for the sleepless nights ahead, although arguably it would be better to let a mother at least start motherhood well rested. A lot of the girls we look after experience insomnia but the good news is that there are some really effective, simple things that may well help break the cycle of sleeplessness and enable you to get the good night's sleep you need.

Tips for sleeping well

- **Develop a bedtime routine.** This will subconsciously prepare the body for sleep. Avoid doing anything stimulating but instead have a bath or do some reading (the more boring your choice of material, the more soporific!) Best of all, have sex; post-coital sleeps are often the best. Going to bed and getting up at the same time, even on the weekends, will create a routine, which most adults (and babies) tend to thrive on.

- **Reserve your bedroom for sleep (and sex).** If you're used to working, sorting or using your phone in bed, it will become a less restful environment for you. Make sure your room is the right temperature (most people sleep better in slightly colder environments) with plenty of fresh air, and if you find you're being woken by light or noise use earplugs and an eye mask.

- **Avoid technology too late in the evening.** Make the bedroom a smartphone- and computer-free zone. Not only is this probably beneficial for your relationship, but evidence shows that using computers and devices with screens late in the evening has a negative impact on sleep.

- **Don't eat a heavy meal just before you go to bed.** Try to keep your evening meal light and if necessary have a small snack before bed; going to bed on an empty stomach can be as counterproductive as going to bed on a very full stomach.

- **Avoid caffeine and stimulants** for at least six hours before bedtime; coffee and chocolate are sleep killers.

- **Exercise generally promotes good sleep** so try to include this in your day, although not too close to bedtime as the endorphins released when you exercise can interfere with good sleep.

- **Try to get plenty of fresh air and natural light during the day.** Even from the beginning of pregnancy, frequent trips to the loo can interrupt sleep. Drink plenty during the day but try to drink less after 6pm to avoid constant loo trips.

- **Don't go to bed until you're tired.** Often the frustration of tossing and turning will preclude sleep. Bear in mind that you might need less sleep than you think, so judge your need for sleep on how you feel rather than the amount of hours you think you've had. Having a nap during the day is crucial if you're tired, but make sure you don't nap after 3pm. Try to avoid a catnap on the sofa in the evening; even a 10-minute doze can stop you going to sleep properly.

- **Try breathing and visualisation exercises.** If you choose to use hypnotherapy as part of your birth preparation (see page 121), the techniques for relaxation can really help you sleep. When you have a lot on your mind these techniques are great for clearing your head. These skills can be learnt at any time.

- **Try quiet and relaxing music or radio.** Avoid listening to anything stimulating. The aim is to distract your mind from your day-to-day worries so that sleep will take over.

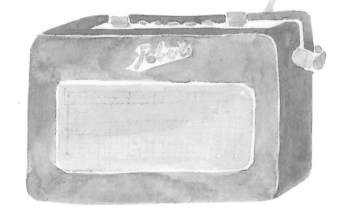

- **Try listening to white noise.** If noises outside are waking you up, having white noise in the room will often drown out external noises.

Getting comfortable in bed

As you get bigger, lying down for long periods of time becomes uncomfortable.
If you're finding that your hips or pressure points are getting sore (due to the
extra weight), try making your bed softer by using a soft mattress topper, or
simply a spare duvet (or two) under your sheet. You might feel more comfortable
if your bump and body have extra support. Many women find specially designed
pregnancy pillows a real help, but otherwise another
spare duvet or pillows tucked around your bump
and back are really effective.

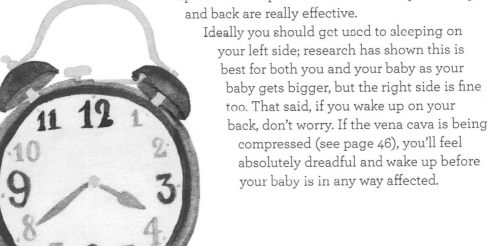

Ideally you should get used to sleeping on
your left side; research has shown this is
best for both you and your baby as your
baby gets bigger, but the right side is fine
too. That said, if you wake up on your
back, don't worry. If the vena cava is being
compressed (see page 46), you'll feel
absolutely dreadful and wake up before
your baby is in any way affected.

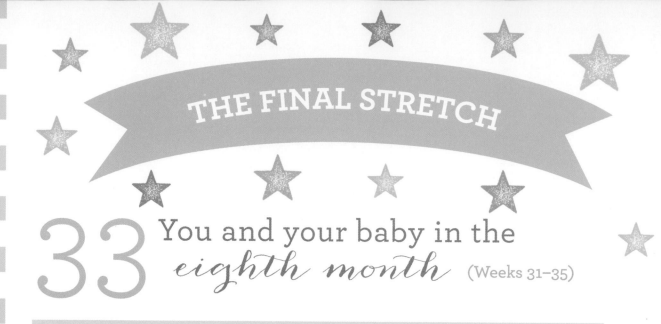

THE FINAL STRETCH

33 You and your baby in the *eighth month* (Weeks 31–35)

You're definitely on the home straight now. The final months of pregnancy can be the hardest, but you're about to get the best present in the world.

In these last few months most mothers put on about 5 kg (11 lb). Your abdomen now has to accommodate up to three times what it is used to and the result can be testing. You might suffer from flatulence, bloating, constipation, shortness of breath, clumsiness, forgetfulness and frequent urination. It is no surprise that women tend to be slightly fragile from this stage. Try to keep your spirits up; the end is in sight.

How you may be feeling

- Whether you like it or not, you will need to slow down. Pregnancy will start to take a real toll on your body. You may start getting backache and develop significant swelling, particularly of your hands and feet. As the fatigue sets in, this is a good opportunity to start listening to your body; ask for help lifting, treat yourself to a taxi, accept favours from friends and generally stop being a superwoman. No matter how busy you are, try to put your feet up and rest during the day, even just for half an hour; you will reap the rewards.
- You may feel pain under your ribs as your uterus is pushing up, and your baby is probably giving you a good old kick in that area as well. If you have significant or persistent pain, go and see a woman's health physiotherapist.
- You will begin to have more frequent antenatal check-ups, and your doctor or midwife will want to be checking the baby's position, size, heartbeat and your blood pressure and urine for any signs of pre-eclampsia.
- You may also be offered a blood test at around 32 weeks to check for anaemia.

- If you are rhesus negative (see page 49) you will need another anti-D injection at around 34 weeks.
- You may also have a late scan if there is any concern about the size or position of the baby or the position of the placenta. If there aren't any concerns but you're curious, you can pay for a late scan privately.

Your baby

As your baby grows and there is less room for her to move, so her movements change. Most women notice a reduction in the number of fetal movements at this stage, although they should still be regular. As she begins to get quite big for your uterus you might well see your bump making the most extraordinary movements!

Your baby's organs are pretty much fully developed now, except for her lungs, which will be ready for action at around 36 weeks. Between 30 and 35 weeks the lungs are maturing incredibly fast but a baby born before 36 weeks will probably still need a little help breathing. Her brain and nervous system are fully developed and her bones (with the exception of her skull) are hardening up. She just has a bit more growing to do. She is still covered in the white waxy substance called vernix, which is protecting her skin and keeping her warm, but the downy lanugo hair is beginning to shed. If you are having a boy, his testicles will descend down from his abdomen into his scrotum around this time.

By 35 weeks your baby probably weighs around 2.3 kg (5 lb) and is about 46 cm (18 inches) long.

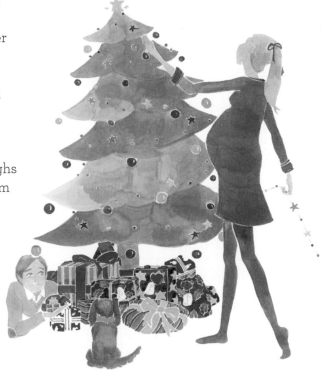

Creating a birth plan

At around this month, you will be encouraged by your healthcare team to write a birth plan. A lot of girls we meet are very worried about what choices to make, how it should be presented and how to make sure their midwife follows it. There is actually a running joke among midwives that the longer and more meticulous the birth plan, the more likely it is not to go to plan. The importance of a birth plan is not the plan itself, but the knowledge you gain from researching it. It's crucial that pregnant women understand the physiology of labour and what options are available to them, but we really discourage women from making a definitive plan per se as, if labour doesn't go to plan, they tend to be disappointed.

A sensible attitude to your birth plan might be as follows:

> ## My birth plan
>
> 'In an ideal world I would like to give birth in a birth pool with Enya playing, the lights dimmed and my husband affectionately stroking my head and whispering gentle words of encouragement into my ear. However since I've not experienced labour and I don't know how long mine will be and how it's going to affect me, nor do I know what position my baby will be in, I'd like the midwives to encourage me to follow my birth plan, but if at any stage either they or I feel that it's not right – maybe for the safety of me and my baby, or that I've simply had enough – we will all agree on another route.'

With this in mind, at this stage in your pregnancy, it's worth thinking about how you would like to give birth, what facilities the hospital or birth centre offers and how they might help you. You need to know about labour and your options before you get there, so by this stage you should be reading and understanding all the chapters up to Chapter 50.

34 Baby *kit*

Shopping for your baby is one of the few really fun parts of pregnancy. While it's true the shops don't shut after your baby is born, it's definitely worth spending the time working out what you need and making sure you've got what you need before your baby is born.

Preparing for the arrival of a baby is an expensive business, and many of the things you need will only be used for a relatively short time. Do ask friends or relatives if they have anything you can borrow and look at second-hand websites, as there are often hardly used items at a fraction of their retail price. It is best to buy new mattresses and car seats but if you do get them second hand, it is essential that they are from a trusted source. The safety of a car seat can be compromised if it has been in a crash or damaged, and because damage might not be outwardly visible, you need to know who it's come from. It's always better to have a clean mattress that you know doesn't have mould spores or dust mites and that is clean.

We can't tell you which buggy to buy; there are hundreds on the market, each filling a specific purpose and suitable for different needs. However, they tend to be big investments so make sure you spend time choosing the one that will be most suitable for you. Think carefully about how you're going to use it. Consider how often will you need to fold and lift it and whether it will fit folded into the back of your car. Will it fit in your hallway and where will it store inside the house? Don't be seduced by trendy denim covers or a leather handle. Once you're a mother, the buggy will be entirely practical and, unless it makes your life easier, you will resent it. There are lots of second-hand buggies in great condition around that can save you a lot of money.

Bedding

Essentials
- 2 sleeping bags (it's best to buy two in case one gets peed, pooed or vomited on)
- 2 swaddling blankets ● At least 2 fitted Moses basket sheets
- At least 2 fitted cot sheets ● 1-2 waterproof mattress protectors
- At least 10 muslins ● At least 1 cellular blanket

Useful but not essential
- 1 summer sleeping bag

Maybe useful
- Woollen blanket (for use in winter, for outside only)

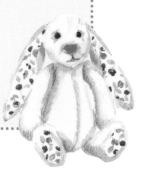

 ## Toys

Essentials
- Bouncy chair

Useful but not essential
- Sheepskin floor mat

Maybe useful
- Baby gym ● Cot mobile
- Comfort toy or blanket

 ## Travelling

Essentials
- Travel cot ● Sheets for travel cot

Useful but not essential
- Travel blackout blind

Maybe useful
- Mattress for travel cot

Nursery

Essentials
- Moses basket and mattress (a stand for this is useful if you've got dogs, cats or small children in the house)
- Cot/cot bed and mattress
- Changing mat

Useful but not essential
- Changing mat covers (you will need a few as they get peed on)
- Nappy bin ● Changing table
- Fan/portable air conditioner

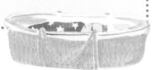

 ## Baby toiletries

Essentials
- Nappy cream ● Baby nail scissors/clippers
- Bowl for topping and tailing
- Baby hairbrush ● Cotton wool
- Cotton buds (for umbilical stump)
- Nappies (start with size 1) ● Nappy bags
- Anti-bacterial clothes soak (such as Napisan)
- Anti-bacterial hand wash or gel

Useful but not essential
- Massage oil

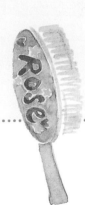

⭐ Out and about

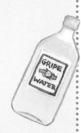

Essentials
- *Pram/buggy*
- *Car seat (legally your baby needs to be in a car seat whenever in a car)*

Useful but not essential
- *Foot muff* ● *Buggy bag clips*
- *Baby carrier/sling* ● *Portable baby changing kit*
- *Sunshade for prams and/or car windows*

Maybe useful
- *Baby-view mirror for car* ● *Sheepskin liner for pram*
- *Isofix base for car seat*

 ## ⭐ Bathtime

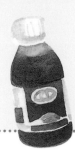

Essentials
- *Plastic bath seat with suction pads*
- *2 sponges – 1 for 'topping' and 1 for 'tailing' (see page 183)*
- *2 bath towels* ● *Baby shampoo/wash*

Useful but not essential
- *Bath toys for older babies*

 ## ⭐ Safety

Essentials
- *Baby monitor (it's useful to get one that monitors the temperature too)*
- *Stair gate (only when they start crawling)*
- *Carbon monoxide detector*
- *Smoke alarms (test regularly)* ● *Fire blanket*

Maybe useful
- *Breathing alarm*

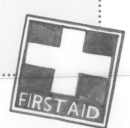

Baby clothes

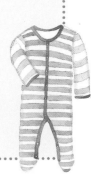

Essentials
- *1 cotton hat* ● *10 cotton bibs*
- *6 short-sleeved vests*
- *6 full-body baby grows with feet and scratch mitts*
- *3 long-sleeved vests (for winter babies)*
- *1 woollen hat (for winter babies only)*
- *2 cardigans (wool for winter, cotton for summer)*

Useful but not essential
- *2 nightgowns (easier for night-time nappy changes)*
- *Outdoor suit (for winter babies)*

See also pages 219–21 on dressing your baby for further advice on clothing.

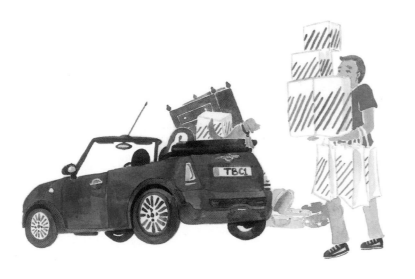

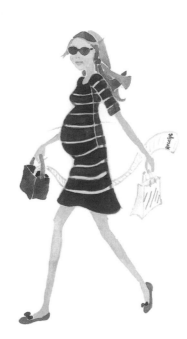

35 Medical kit for you *and your baby*

I know I am a doctor but, nonetheless, I truly think that having a medical kit, which you have put together before the arrival of your family, will not be something that you will ever regret. Yes, you can probably always go out and buy items when you need them but that does not help you when it is 3am and you have a baby with a fever or a bee has just stung your child! Hopefully you won't have to use it much in the early days, but the likelihood is that you will use it as your baby gets older and is more likely to injure herself and become ill. There is no doubt that being prepared makes motherhood a little bit easier ...

Essential advice on using medicines

Please note that babies are very sensitive to medications. You should always take care to thoroughly read any labels to make sure products are suitable for your baby. Even 'infant' products are often for babies over a certain age only, so please check any age recommendations. If you have any doubt about using a medication or product, seek advice from your GP.

Please remember that you should always seek medical advice before treating your child. Having a first-aid kit is useful to have in the house but if your child is unwell or injured you should see a medical professional.

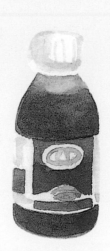

'What kind of thermometer is best for my baby?'
This is a piece of kit that you will use a lot with children in the house and it is worth investing in a good one that allows you to take their temperature with ease. If your baby is ill and you speak to a doctor, the first thing they will ask is what her temperature is. Similarly if your baby is off-colour, it is reassuring to know she doesn't have a temperature. A thermometer is also a great piece of kit for you in your pregnancy, as having a temperature is an indication of infection, which needs to be treated as soon as possible.

Most doctors use 'ear thermometers'; if you want one of these you should ensure it is one of the top-of-the-range ones as the cheaper ones are not very accurate. Ear thermometers are especially good for babies as you can take their temperature in their sleep without waking them.

 ## What you should have in your medical kit

Basics
- Thermometer
- First-aid manual

General medicines
- Infant paracetamol, such as Calpol
- Infant ibuprofen, such as Nurofen for Children
- Colic-relief treatment, such as Infacol or Gripe water
- Teething granules, such as Chamomilla 200 c
- Oral-rehydration solution, such as Dioralyte

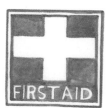

For colds, congestion and coughs
- Saline nasal spray
- Nasal aspirator
- Decongestant drops, such as Karvol or Olbas oil
- Chest rub for babies
- Humidifier (anecdotally this can alleviate coughing at night)

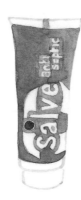

For cuts, bruises and burns
- It's worth buying an over-the-counter first-aid kit, which contains bandages, dressings, tape, scissors, etc.
- Antiseptic spray, such as Savlon
- Plasters
- Ice pack
- Cotton wool
- Saline solution pods
- Sterile eyewash
- Tweezers
- Hand sanitiser
- Arnica (cream and tablets)
- Burn cream

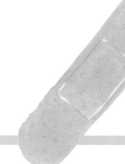

For bites or allergic reactions
- Wasp spray, such as Wasp-Eze
- Infant antihistamine, such as Piriton Allergy Syrup
- Children's mosquito repellent
- Antihistamine cream
- Local anaesthetic spray or 'cold spray' for bites and stings

---

First aid

It is really important that you do a paediatric first-aid course before your baby arrives so that, at the bare minimum, you know how to recognise a medical emergency and resuscitate a newborn. It will also stand you in good stead for dealing with accidents and emergencies as your child grows. Your partner and anyone else who might be looking after your child should also have paediatric first-aid training and know what to do if a child is choking or how to do basic life support for a newborn or child; it can be the difference between life and death.

36 Starting to prepare for the *arrival of your baby*

At some point in your last trimester it's worth taking some time to think about the practicalities of your baby's arrival. One mother described coming home as 'being given the most precious thing in the world and realising that it doesn't come with any operating instructions'.

You will most likely return from hospital exhausted, overwhelmed and emotional, so if there is any chance of getting some help at home, take it.

 ## What will you need help with?

- **Cooking:** The last thing you'll feel like doing is slaving over a hot stove, but the likelihood is that after labour you probably won't have eaten much over the last few days, so you'll be in dire need of a nutritious and substantial meal. If a friend or family member offers to do some cooking, take them up on the offer. However, if that is not an option, you can either fill your freezer with nutritious shop-bought ready meals or spend some time before your baby is born preparing home-cooked meals that can be frozen.

- **Cleaning:** You're going to be sore after your baby is born and the last thing you should be doing is changing sheets or hoovering.

- **Washing:** Nothing will prepare you for the mountains of washing. Babies are sick and poo a lot and as a result need a lot of clothing changes. The same goes for you (well hopefully not the sick and the poo); you'll probably want to change your pyjamas every day and possibly even your bedding due to getting sweaty at night (see page 178).

- **Building confidence:** Every new parent feels entirely unqualified to look after their babies and, while they aren't, it's nice to have someone whose advice you can ask. This is when grandmothers really come into their own; remember they've done it before.

- **Company:** Being a new mother can be a lonely business. It involves hours upon hours of the same feeding, winding, nappy changing, settling, feeding, winding, nappy changing, settling ... routine. As amazing as spending time with your newborn is, it's great to have some adult conversation mixed in. Having someone or a rota of people coming to help and spend a few hours with you every day will lift your spirits.

> *'When my daughter was born my friend Susan popped around with three days' worth of pre-cooked food for me. It was the best baby present I ever got. I didn't have to think, shop, prepare or cook; I just devoured.'* ALEX, BUMP CLASS

What type of help is available

- **Fathers:** In the UK, fathers are entitled to take two weeks of 'ordinary' paternity leave (and can now take 'additional' paternity leave if their partner returns to work before 12 months). It's crucial for a father to take some time to get to know his baby and support his family, so ensure he actually takes some leave and encourage him to be hands-on during this time.

- **Parents and family members:** Many girls find that their relationship with their mother changes hugely after they've given birth; the reality of the struggles of motherhood gives them a newfound respect for what their mother has achieved. New mothers really need to be mothered themselves and it's no bad idea if a parent or family member can come and spend some time with you – helping with the baby, helping around the house and, having done it before, bringing you valuable experience and building your confidence.

- **Postnatal doula:** Paid by the hour, these wonderful ladies are a general help to new mothers. As well as helping with the baby, they cook, clean, help and advise, look after the mother and help with any other children. Although they might be a mother themselves and might have done a course, there is no actual qualification needed to become a doula, so make sure you get a recommendation or go through a doula organisation.

- **Maternity nurse:** These are essentially nannies (not nurses) who specialise in looking after newborn babies and supporting mothers. They generally live with you, either in the baby's room or in their own space, and charge for every 24 hours. Their role is essentially looking after the baby and mother, including 'nursery duties', such as doing the baby's washing, sterilising, feeding, etc. It's important that you clarify their role before they start. Over the time she is with you, a good maternity nurse should teach you how to look after your baby, encourage and help with feeding (either breast or bottle). They often sleep in the same room as the baby, bringing her to you for feeding and then taking her away to be winded and settled, allowing you precious extra sleep.

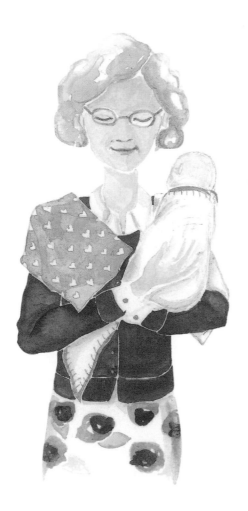

Having a maternity nurse is a huge help but they are expensive. Historically they were called 'monthly nurses' and stayed for the first month of the baby's life but nowadays they're more flexible and are generally happy to help for as little as a week. They can even come for shorter periods as the baby gets older to help with troubleshooting and helping with any sleep issues.

- **Night nannies:** These nannies will come for a 12-hour shift, usually around 7pm to 7am to look after the baby during the night. As they're only coming for the night, they won't do any other nursery duties. For some people, who prefer to be on their own during the day, a night nanny is a great option, allowing them to have a decent night's sleep, although the price difference between a night nanny and a 24-hour maternity nurse is often negligible. Night nannies are very flexible; they can come for a few nights a week or a longer stint. As with maternity nurses, they can also come occasionally as the baby gets older to help with any issues.

Currently in the UK anyone can call themselves a maternity nurse, night nanny or doula, so make sure you check their references thoroughly and ensure they are DBS/CRB-checked and that their first-aid training is up to date.

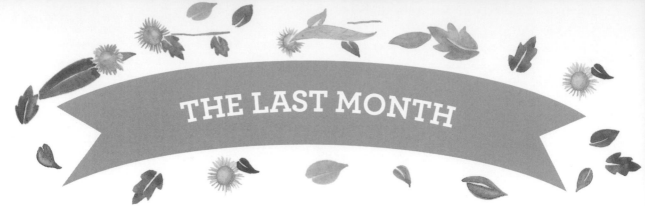

THE LAST MONTH

37 You and your baby in the *ninth month* (Weeks 36–40)

A lot of women feel that pregnancy is a month too long and by the time they get to 36 weeks they're fed up and desperate to meet the little person they've been growing. Your baby is considered term from 37 weeks, so by then you should be ready for her arrival. That said, every extra week she has been growing inside you is beneficial, so control your excitement and anticipation and focus on your last weeks of being able to relax.

You might want to consider paying for a screening test for the bacteria Group B Streptococcus at this point. See page 129 for further details.

 ### How you may be feeling

- You are likely to feel tired and fed up – every movement might feel an effort.
- You should have started your maternity leave by now and you probably will find that you have a strong nesting instinct, wanting to make everything perfect for the arrival of your baby. Try not to overdo it. You really don't need to iron every muslin square or hoover the nursery for the fourth time. However, it is important to feel prepared so that you can relax and wait for the arrival of your baby.
- The hormone changes occurring later in the pregnancy will cause your breasts to swell (even more!), and you may start producing small amounts of the first breast milk, colostrum. This can leak at unexpected times, for example if you hear a baby crying or when you are having sex. You may also notice an increased vaginal discharge.
- You will probably be feeling very tired and may well be having problems sleeping, perhaps continually being woken by discomfort or needing to empty your bladder.

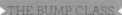

● At some point in this last month it is common to feel your baby's head gradually drop lower down into the pelvis and become 'engaged'. When this happens your bump measurement may reduce a bit and you will feel less pressure against your ribs and diaphragm. However, once your baby is engaged, you might feel more pressure on your bladder and perineum – some women have the sensation their baby is going to fall out. Don't worry. This is a normal sensation and it won't just fall out. However, don't be too concerned about how 'engaged' your baby is and when this happens. For some women it happens some weeks before labour starts and for some their baby does not 'drop' until their labour has started.

TIP
As your due date approaches, it's worth speaking to a homeopathist about taking arnica, which is said to help with bruising after birth. It might be something that you should be taking before the delivery or at the onset of labour to have the maximum effect.

Your baby

Your baby (including her lungs) is now fully cooked and ready for the outside world. Her intestine is fully formed and contains a dark green sticky substance called 'meconium', which is passed as your baby's first poo.

> **'What is meconium?'**
> Meconium consists of secretions from your baby's bowel, gall bladder and liver, as well as dead skin cells and the remains of the hair that was initially covering the baby, the lanugo.

In this last month your midwife will check how engaged your baby is by determining how much of her head they can feel before it emerges into the pelvis. To measure this, midwives assess how many 'fifths' of your baby's head they can feel. So, if they can feel three-fifths of your baby's head in your abdomen, it is three-fifths 'palpable' or two-fifths 'engaged'.

After 36 weeks, if your baby is not head down, it is much less likely to change position because of the limited space, so the team looking after you will want to discuss the possibility of trying to turn the baby (see box on next page).

'What if my baby is breech?'

When a baby is 'breech' it means her head is up, with her bottom sitting in the pelvis. If the baby is breech at 35 weeks there is still a chance that she may turn head down spontaneously. However, by 37 weeks this is unlikely.

You may be offered an ECV (external cephalic version), which is when an obstetrician attempts to turn the baby using gentle sustained pressure. This should always be done in hospital with appropriate monitoring. It is successful in 50–60 per cent of cases.

Although vaginal breech deliveries are possible, studies have shown that the safest way to deliver a breech baby is by caesarean section.

There is some (limited) evidence that acupuncture and moxibustion (an ancient Chinese technique of burning herbs and stimulating acupressure points) may help turn the baby.

Most babies at 40 weeks weigh around 3.5 kg (8 lb), although it is common for little boys to weigh more than little girls. The average head-to-toe length is 50 cm (20 inches), and the crown-to-rump length is about 38 cm (15 inches).

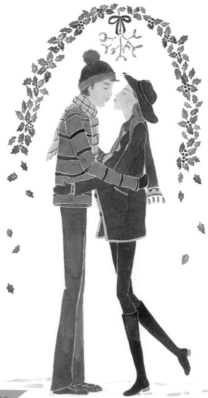

38 Preparing to be *a mother*

You are probably guilty of what is common among most mothers – only thinking about your baby. As important as your baby is, it's worth spending a little time preparing yourself for motherhood. Having a baby is a big deal and you need to be looked after just as much as your baby does.

 ## Perineal massage

So many pregnant girls are scared of tearing or episiotomy (see page 140) during birth. Research has shown that doing perineal massage for three to five weeks before your delivery can reduce the chances of these. It will not eliminate the chances, but most girls are happy to do anything that might help. Essentially massaging the perineum (the tissue between the back wall of the vagina and the back passage) with a degree of pressure will stretch it in preparation for the birth.

Here are simple steps for perineal massage:

1. Lie down on your side and insert one or both thumbs into the back of the vagina.
2. Use a natural, unscented oil as a lubricant (an olive or sunflower oil that you have in your kitchen will do just fine).
3. Gently but firmly massage the perineal tissue for 5–10 minutes at a time.
4. It should not be painful but you might feel a stinging, stretching sensation, which is similar to what you will feel pushing your baby out.

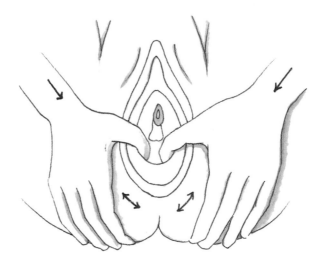

'I used the Epi-no in my pregnancy – essentially a balloon that you insert into your vagina and pump up, slowly stretching the tissue. Over three weeks you gradually pump it up more and more until you get to 10 cm, the size of the average baby's head. There have not yet been any good studies to suggest this makes birth any easier but, from a psychological point of view, it gave me the confidence to know I could fit a baby through there. My feeling was that, from an unscientific point of view, it makes total sense. I've never been able to touch my toes and if someone forced me to I could, but I would probably damage my back in the process. If I had three weeks to slowly stretch, I'd achieve the same thing, without the damage.' MARINA

Post-birth clothes

Once your baby is born, a major part of your role is essentially that of a feeding machine, and dealing with this successfully requires a degree of preparation. Breastfeeding bras are a must. At 37 weeks you need to get measured. Once your milk comes in your breasts will grow considerably so these bras will be bigger than you anticipate. We recommend you buy at least four as they get mucky and sweaty, and you'll want to change them frequently.

If you're planning to breastfeed, breastfeeding tops make the whole process much more discreet. They have a clever opening allowing you to breastfeed without exposing your whole (usually very large, veiny) breast. They're easy to find online so it's worth investing in a handful of these before your baby comes.

Remember that, once your baby is born, you will still look about six months pregnant. Although your tummy does go down quickly, most women continue to wear their maternity clothes for some weeks, if not months. Stretchy trousers and leggings are great for the post-birth period – concentrate on comfort rather than style for the first few weeks.

You will bleed for four to six weeks after your baby is born, regardless of whether you've had a caesarean or a natural birth (see page 163), and this will initially be much more significant than a period. Normal sanitary pads will be inadequate, so buy plenty of maternity pads (be prepared: they're thick). We even recommend using incontinence pants at night for the first few days to prevent leakage in bed.

Shopping list for new mums

- 4 nursing bras
- 2 nursing nighties
- Breast pads
- Nipple cream
- Nipple shields
- Feeding tops
- Feeding scarf
- Stretchy trousers
- Cooling gel pad for your perineum (such as a Femé pad)
- 20 pairs of disposable knickers
- Incontinence pants (useful for immediately after birth or the first few nights)
- Maternity pads
- Pack of 6 waterproof pads to go under your sheets

Q&A

'Is it "courteous" to the midwives and doctors to "tidy up down there"?'
Whether or not women should wax or shave before birth is one of the most commonly asked questions in our all-girls groups, and the answer, quite honestly, from every midwife and doctor we've asked is no! These professionals are used to seeing this part of our anatomy on a daily basis – for them it's like looking at a computer screen. Most women are hairy; it's what's natural and the way most women choose to be.

If 'tidying up' is something that will make you feel more comfortable, then by all means go ahead. However, bear in mind that some women find regrowth after a wax quite itchy and uncomfortable and, believe us, this is the last thing you need when you have a sore perineum after birth. We generally advise girls not to worry, and instead to spend the money and time on a nice relaxing massage!

39 What to pack in your *labour bag*

You should have packed the bag you will take to hospital by 37 weeks. By this time your baby is term and if born would not be considered premature. The suggested list below will seem like a lot to pack, but we've thought really carefully about what helps women in labour. As you'll be reminded again and again as a mother, it's best to be very well prepared.

It's worth taking two bags: one for labour (which is hot, sweaty and messy) and one bag for after it's all over – when you've showered and can get into nice, clean clothes, which will make you feel human again.

 Labour bag one
- Energy tablets and (non-fizzy) sports drinks (these are great for quick energy boosts and replacing lost minerals and salts)
- Snacks – you're unlikely to eat a great deal but it's important to keep your energy up in labour. Think about taking some snacks for your partner as well – they will need sustenance
- Bottle of water (ideally with sports top) – it's important to stay hydrated by sipping water throughout
- Cooling water spray and/or flannel
- Maternity pads
- Short nightie (preferably cheap as it might get ruined!)
- Hair ties and clips (as you'll want your hair out of your face)
- Music or hypnobirthing CDs and earphones
- Pillow(s) with coloured pillow case(s) so you know it is yours
- Book/iPad or something to do (if you have an epidural)
- Lip balm
- Cheap slippers or flip flops (these are also likely to get ruined)
- TENS machine (see page 122)
- Homeopathic or natural remedies, such as arnica or Rescue Remedy
- Phone and chargers
- Camera
- Cash for parking

Labour bag two

For your baby

(This list assumes you'll stay one night.)

- Set of clothes for baby (2 short-sleeved vests, 2 baby grows, a cardigan, blanket and a hat)
- Newborn or size-1 nappies and cotton wool
- Dummies
- Car seat – you should make sure you know how to put the baby in it and how to fix it into the car

For you

- A comfy nightie with a button-down top for breastfeeding
- A short dressing gown
- 2 breastfeeding bras
- Breast pads
- Nipple cream
- Disposable pants/incontinence pants
- Femé pad (see page 107)
- Nice shower gel, shampoo, body cream and bubble bath
- Antiseptic wipes
- Earplugs and eye mask
- Arnica (it's best to start taking this the week before you're due and continuing for 10 days afterwards to help your body heal)
- Toothbrush and toothpaste
- Some make-up
- Clothes to go home in (these will probably be pregnancy clothes; see page 61)

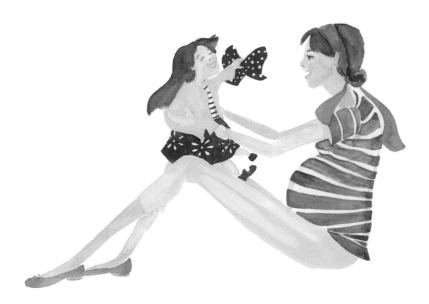

'They say memories are defined by photos. When I had my son, I was counting on my "maternal glow" to ensure the ubiquitous picture would look nice. After a three-day labour, this was not the case. That early photo is so special and I would love to have it framed and up in my house. But there's no way with me looking like I'd spent three days in a war zone! So I'd recommend packing a teeny bit of make-up – more than anything looking halfway decent will make you feel better.' MARINA

Don't forget your hospital notes
It's best to take your hospital notes everywhere with you in your last trimester. If you have to rush into hospital it will make the medical staff's job faster and easier if you have your notes on you.

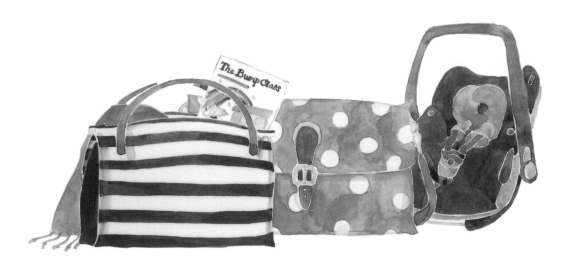

40 Going *overdue*

Although your due date is calculated at 40 weeks, most first-time mothers give birth closer to 41 weeks. Pregnant women vary in their attitudes to going overdue. First-time mothers are often desperate to finally meet their baby and any day after 40 weeks is sheer torture. With second and subsequent pregnancies mothers frequently adopt the view 'easier in than out' and are quite happy to have a week extra putting their feet up before the challenges of looking after a newborn start.

Officially you're term from 37 weeks and most babies are born by 42 weeks. That said, most doctors agree that it is in the baby's best interests to stay inside for as close to 40 weeks as possible unless there is a medical reason not to.

Once you pass 40 weeks, however, the various risks begin to increase and it's common practice to be reviewed regularly and sometimes even scanned. In the NHS it is standard practice to let women go up to 42 weeks but after that you will be encouraged to have an induction, as the risks of continuing the pregnancy greatly outweigh the risks of induction. (See page 114 for information on being induced.)

When you are overdue it is particularly important to monitor your baby's movements, and if you have any concerns you should see your midwife or doctor immediately.

Q&A

'I've heard that it's fine to give birth at 43 weeks – is this right?'
While many babies born at 43 weeks are indeed healthy, to put it into perspective: the risk of stillbirth doubles from 42 to 43 weeks. Most doctors agree that this is good reason for induction to begin at around 41 weeks so that babies are born by 42 weeks.

Natural methods for bringing on labour – fact or fiction?

Most women who go overdue usually are keen to know if there are any natural techniques to kick-start labour. So what works and what doesn't?

- **Curry:** Curry, like castor oil, is quite a good laxative, and clearing out the bowels can be a trigger for labour to start. However, the curry needs to be spicy enough to give you diarrhoea, which many women simply can't face at 40 weeks pregnant.

- **Sex:** Was this dreamt up by sex-starved men or based on fact? Sadly a mid-afternoon quickie will probably not be enough to get labour going. Although sperm does contain prostaglandins, which in high doses soften the cervix, you would need huge amounts of semen to produce anywhere near the same effect as the vaginal gel used in induction! Most women at 40 weeks pregnant would prefer a small pessary to sex 20 times a day …

- **Nipple stimulation:** This causes release of the hormone oxytocin, which stimulates the uterus to contract. A recent study confirmed that nipple stimulation for 1–3 hours increased the chance of going into labour, so if you've got the time, energy and inclination, go for it. However, if contractions start, leave your nipples alone. Beware of making your nipples sore as they've got an important role to play over the coming weeks and months.

- **Raspberry leaf tea, evening primrose oil or pineapple:** These are thought to help soften the cervix and lead to more coordinated contractions. However, recent studies have failed to show any significant benefit both in terms of when labour starts or how quickly it progresses.

- **Membrane sweep:** This is when the midwife attempts to get things going by trying to stretch the cervix and separate it from the membranes containing the baby. This is supposed to stimulate prostaglandin release and trigger labour. Although safe from 38 weeks, it's more effective from 40 weeks and can be quite uncomfortable. Evidence for how effective this is, however, is very tenuous.

- **Acupuncture and reflexology:** Anecdotally we've come across many women who say their labour has been triggered by these. However, it is impossible to know for sure whether their labour would have started anyway, and currently there is no robust evidence to say that it is effective.

THE BUMP CLASS

- **Homeopathy:** A number of homeopathic agents, taken from 36 weeks, are thought to result in a shorter labour, although there is no evidence to support this. If you want to give it a try, get advice from a trusted homeopath.

- **Walking:** Keeping upright and active can help move the baby's head down into a good position for labour. Don't overdo it, but becoming a couch potato will probably not help get labour started.

- **Be relaxed:** Probably the best thing you can do is not get frustrated that labour doesn't seem to be starting. Adopt the view that the baby will come when it's ready and try not to obsess about it.

> *'From experience with my own patients, I have certainly experienced that babies will often be delayed for a few days until the mother is relaxed and ready, and a few studies have suggested that this could well be the case.'* CHIARA

In most cases any kind of 'natural' induction is more successful after 40 weeks, so our advice would be to rest, relax and spoil yourself at the end of your pregnancy.

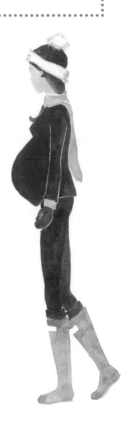

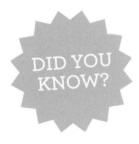

DID YOU KNOW?

Racial background may play a part in when your baby finally arrives. Studies have shown that more South Asian and black women give birth before 39 weeks than white women.

41 Induction

We meet an extraordinary amount of women who are terrified of induction, having heard countless horror stories. There really isn't any need for this fear; induction often just kick-starts labour, which then continues completely naturally. In fact two-thirds of inductions progress without the need for any further medical intervention in the birth.

There are many reasons that your baby might have to be delivered early and it's important that you understand these reasons. A doctor will not base their decision for induction on their convenience; it will always be in your and your baby's best interests. If you are advised to have an induction, start getting excited – you're about to finally meet your baby!

 ## Why you might be induced

- If you are overdue: After 42 weeks the risk of stillbirth doubles (see page 111).
- If your waters break and contractions don't start: Once the waters have broken, the sterile environment of the amniotic sac is compromised and the risk of infection to the baby and mother increases.
- If the baby is not growing well: This may be a sign that your placenta is not working as well as it was (charmingly referred to as an 'ageing placenta').
- If you have high blood pressure or pre-eclampsia: This can develop into eclampsia, which is potentially fatal for the mother.
- If you have gestational diabetes: Babies born to mothers with this are at higher risk of complications and are often also substantially larger, so your obstetrician and midwife will keep a close eye on you and induce if necessary.
- Other medical reasons: There are various other concerns and issues that might mean your doctor or midwife suggests an induction. They will discuss this with you so that you understand the reasons for doing it.

What happens in an induction?

There are three stages to induction but you may well not have to have all three. If at any point your labour starts, they'll let you progress without further intervention, unless it's necessary:

1. Using a vaginal gel, tablet or pessary: These are used to insert prostaglandin into the vagina, which softens the cervix. It normally takes some time to start working and the process may need to be repeated a few times.
2. Breaking the waters: This is also known as artificial rupture of membranes (or ARM). Once the cervix is soft enough and slightly dilated from the gel, the midwife should be able to break the waters. This is done by making a small nick in the sack that is holding the baby in the waters, rather like bursting a water balloon. Most women find it mildly uncomfortable but not excruciating; however, you can use gas and air if you need it.
3. Stimulating the contractions: If your contractions do not start naturally or are not strong enough, you will be given the hormone oxytocin through an intravenous drip. This is the same hormone that your body produces for contractions. The more of the drug you are given the stronger the contractions are so the doctors will monitor the contractions and adjust the dose accordingly. Your contractions and your baby's heart rate will need to be monitored continuously and you will be examined every four hours.

It's important to remember that, although the monitoring and the drip are a bit unwieldy, it is still absolutely possible and important for you to be as mobile and upright as possible and that you can use any of the techniques you had been planning to help you through labour.

TIPS
- When induction starts things may take a while to kick off. Try to rest.
- When labour starts try to use all the techniques you may have planned, no matter where you are. (For example, keeping the room dark, not having too many people, with music on and using breathing and visualisation exercises; see pages 118–22).
- Induced labour can be more painful and you may need an epidural (see page 123). Keep an open mind and don't beat yourself up about this.
- Inductions can feel harder than normal labour so prepare by being patient and trying not to rush it, and make sure you have really good support.

42 Synopsis *of labour*

We like to think about the day you give birth as the only time you'll go on a blind date where you're guaranteed to meet the love of your life. Some girls on The Bump Class cannot wait for their first contraction and others, having been inundated with horror stories, are absolutely terrified. If you fall into the latter category, consider this: if childbirth were really so bad, would we really have a global population explosion? The answer is no; as a breed, we'd be so scared that second children would simply not happen. While it's happening, it can feel brutal, some girls feel out of control and think they can't do it, but when your baby is born, all of those feelings simply disappear and you're left with the greatest gift in the world.

Labour is split into four different stages and – before we start talking about each stage in more detail – it's really important that you have a good overview of the whole process.

Labour is essentially the softening and opening of your cervix, which allows your baby to descend into the birth canal and be born. The cervix is the neck of the womb, which in pregnancy is tightly shut, holding your baby inside. As labour starts, your cervix begins to soften and slowly open, dilating to about 10 cm, which is big enough to deliver your baby.

It's important to remember that all women are different and predicting labour is impossible. Therefore all the timings and details below are based on what happens normally. We all know that there are exceptions so please bear this in mind! In the interest of giving a simple overview of labour, we have generalised here. For a more detailed description of the stages see pages 128–43.

1. **Early labour (or the 'latent stage'):** This is the phase when your cervix is softening and starting to open to 3–4 cm. During this stage you will usually be at home – not because the hospital doesn't want to have you in but because women generally progress better at this stage at home. You will feel contractions but they might be irregular. If they are regular, they usually don't last too long (around 30 seconds to a minute) and there can be anything from 5–15 minutes between them, sometimes even longer.

2. **Active labour:** This is when your cervix is dilating from 4–10 cm. Here your contractions are usually coming regularly at 3–5-minute intervals and lasting longer. This is when most people go to the birth centre or hospital, or, if they're giving birth at home, when their midwife should be with them. Once you're in active labour, there should be a dedicated midwife with you until you deliver your baby. This stage usually lasts anywhere between 6 and 18 hours with first-time mothers – usually at the longer end of the spectrum.

3. **Pushing:** This is when you push your baby out. Contractions are very intense and last even longer, with a shorter interval in between them, but the good news is that this stage usually lasts no longer than 1–2 hours.

4. **The delivery of the placenta.**

*Never say never – these timings are just a guide and are based on the majority of labours.

Stage	Dilation	Contractions	Approximate* duration
Early labour	Cervix softening and dilating to 3–4 cm	Sometimes irregular or 5–15 minutes apart	Anything up to 3 days
Active labour/ Established labour	4–10 cm	Regular, 3–5 minutes apart	6–18 hours
Pushing		Intense, close together	1–2 hours
Delivery of the placenta		Less intense but noticeable	5–60 minutes

43 Pain relief *in labour*

Every woman approaches her labour differently. For some an epidural at the earliest possible opportunity is what they want. Others are adamant not to use any forms of medicalised pain relief for what is essentially a natural process. No matter what your initial plans are, it's important to realise that every woman feels the pain of labour in a different way. What we advise is to have an open mind.

There are all sorts of factors that will determine the type of pain relief you might use, such as:

- The length of your labour
- The position of your baby
- The size of your baby
- The shape of your pelvis
- How relaxed you feel in your birth environment
- How much you've practised relaxation techniques or hypnosis
- Your wishes for pain relief

The type of pain relief you end up using has absolutely no bearing on how well you've done in labour or your future abilities as a mother. For many women it's not the intensity of contractions that leads them to have an epidural but the fact that they are exhausted after some days of contractions. We encourage every woman to go into labour with an open mind about the kind of pain relief they might need, but armed with the knowledge of what is available to them.

⭐ Natural pain-relief techniques

Whatever your preference, we encourage every girl to investigate techniques that have helped millions of women giving birth for centuries. If you can use one or a combination of the below to help you through even just the latent stage, the time investment will have been worth it. We've seen women banking on an epidural who have been amazed at how well water and hypnotherapy have got them through their whole labour.

Distraction: Some women find distraction a great form of pain relief in early labour. Music, cooking, going for a walk, household chores and funny films (avoid emotional ones) are brilliant forms of distraction.

Massage: While some women hate to be touched in labour, others find touch and massage great for easing the discomfort. Hard massage in the lower back is a firm favourite, but be guided by what you feel like at the time.

Breathing: This is something you have to practise in the build-up to your labour. Studies have shown that if you maintain slow, deep breaths (in through your nose and out through your mouth) during your contractions, not only is the pain less intense but the contractions are less exhausting over time. Breathing is also a great way of reducing anxiety.

How to breathe through your contractions

- Remember to keep your breathing slow, deep and rhythmic.
- Focus on keeping your muscles relaxed, especially your jaw, shoulders and pelvic floor.
- Breathe in through your nose and out through your mouth.
- Practise your breathing in your pregnancy and ask your birthing partner to help you.
- Try to count during your breaths and set a target – say up to six on your way in and ten on your way out.
- Or try just saying the word 'RE ... LAX' very slowly: the 're–' as you breathe in and the '–lax' as you breathe out.

'I focused on my breathing before my labour and it really helped me through my contractions. Towards the end, as I got tired, I did need to be reminded to keep my breathing steady. I ended up having an emergency caesarean and, understandably, I was quite anxious. I found that controlling my breathing really helped me to stay calm during the operation and, to be honest, it's something I continue to use in everyday life – from when my baby is crying in the car to when I get nervous flying. I'm amazed by how much simple breathing even now helps me control my anxiety, stress levels and even pain.'
LAURA, BUMP CLASS

Visualisation: Your state of mind is so important in labour. Try to visualise a safe and secure place with happy memories.

Water (shower or bath at home): Water is a brilliant form of pain relief in early labour; women we encounter every day swear by this simple method. You should make sure your bump is totally immersed in water. The temperature shouldn't be too hot to make you sweat, but be sure to keep on topping it up so that it doesn't become tepid. A warm shower concentrated on the parts where the pain is most intense will help.

Birthing pool: Just as a bath or shower in early labour can help with pain, so can a birthing pool once you're in established labour. These pools are designed so that women can be upright and mobile in the water while benefitting from the relative weightlessness that water gives you. As long as there are no concerns about your progress, there is no time limit for being in the pool. While some women prefer to get out of the water to actually deliver their baby (it really depends on what you feel at the time), many babies are actually born in the water.

'Is it safe to give birth in a birthing pool?'

Many mothers worry that being born into water would carry a risk of their baby 'drowning'. However, remember your baby is coming from water (amniotic fluid) and the stimulus to breathe is generally only through hitting the cold air or being handled. The pool is kept at exactly the right temperature (your body temperature) and the midwife will handle your baby as little as possible as she's being born. The midwife will usually deliver the baby and hand her up to the mother between her legs. The mother lifts the baby out of the water and onto her chest. As long as you have fully trained midwives supporting you in water birth, this is a safe and wonderful birth method both for mother and baby.

If the midwives are at all concerned, they will recommend that you get out of the water. If you've got your heart set on a water birth, remember they'll only recommend this if it's best for your and your baby's well-being. By all means understand why they are recommending this, but, instead of feeling disappointed, focus instead on the fact that, however it happens, the moment you meet your baby is utterly magical.

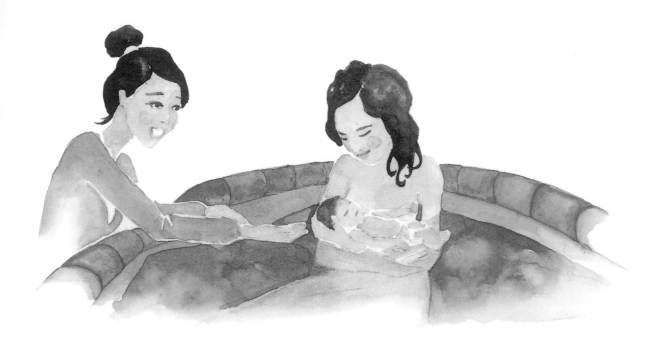

Hypnosis (hypnobirthing): There is a theory that we all have a tendency to panic once labour starts and go into 'fight or flight' mode. By using self-hypnosis it's possible to overcome this anxiety and remain relaxed. The concept is that when fear is replaced by relaxation, the fear chemical (adrenaline) is replaced by increased amounts of oxytocin, prostaglandin and endorphins. These labour hormones will relax the muscles, making labour easier, often quicker and less painful. Hypnosis isn't for everyone, but if you're keen to give it a try you do need to be prepared to really invest some time in it. You can't expect to listen to a CD once and sail through labour by hypnosis. The more time you take to really hone your skill, the more likely you are to really benefit from this technique.

Birth environment: Don't underestimate the importance of your birth environment. If a woman does not feel secure and happy, labour might well slow down. This is so often seen when women go into hospital – their labour has been progressing well at home, but slows down once they arrive in the more intimidating environment. If you do have a change in environment, either going into hospital or a birth centre, we advise you to try to take yourself into your own little world and focus just on your labour rather than what is going on around you. Put some headphones on, close your eyes and try to use visualisation during the transfer. Once in your room, don't be afraid to make it your own. Turn down the lights, make it smell

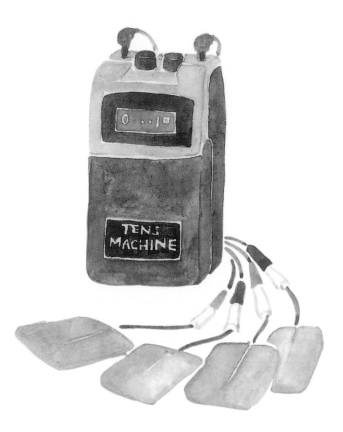

nice with a flameless oil burner and put some music on. It's fine to ask the midwives to keep disturbance to a minimum if you're coping well.

TENS machine: This little machine really helps a lot of women – some for a part and some all the way through labour. It is based on the theory that small electrical pulses affect the way pain signals are sent to the brain, therefore reducing the pain. You can rent or buy a small machine that sends electrical pulses to the back through sticky pads. While you're having a contraction you use a boost button to activate the pulses. Make sure you get one specifically for pregnancy as they're also used for other types of pain.

 Medical pain-relief options

Paracetamol: People underestimate humble paracetamol but a normal dose (1,000 mg) of paracetamol, taken regularly every 6 hours can provide a really good baseline pain relief. However, it is no good taking one every so often; the real benefit will be derived from the maximum dose every 4–6 hours.

Gas and air: Otherwise known as nitrous oxide or laughing gas, this gas will often take the edge off contractions. Available on labour wards and birth centres, as well as for home births, it is breathed through a mouthpiece and can be a great pain reliever.

How to use gas and air
- It takes a few moments for the effects to build up so the key is to start breathing it as soon as you start to feel the contraction so that it is most effective when the contraction is at its peak.
- As soon as you start to feel anything that could be a contraction, take long, deep breaths through the mouthpiece.
- Once your contraction is on the way out, you can stop breathing the gas and air.

It can make some women feel sick in the early stages but if you persevere that feeling will usually go and it's worth it!

Pethidine/diamorphine: An injection of an opiate can be given in labour for women who simply aren't coping with the pain. The injection will make you sleepy and, while it won't take the pain away completely, it will take the edge off your contractions, allowing you to rest. We wouldn't suggest having this too close to the end of your labour as many women say they felt slightly out of it when their baby was born. It also passes through the placenta to the baby and, while it won't cause any long-term effects, babies are often born sleepy and may not feed so well initially.

Epidural: This is the only form of pain relief that will totally take the pain of labour away. Always administered by an anaesthetist, local anaesthetic is injected through the back into the spinal fluid via a small flexible plastic tube and topped up when needed. See the next chapter for a fuller discussion of the pros and cons of this form of pain relief.

'Many women do wonder why anyone wants to go through labour without an epidural! But there are many benefits if this is a possibility. If you are looked after by a midwife (preferably in a birth centre) and avoid an epidural, then you are more likely to have fewer medical procedures, such as a drip, a catheter or an episiotomy. Also, most birth centres have a private room for you, your baby and your partner after the birth. You can usually go home directly from there if all is well. This allows your new family to bond in the first hours away from the communal ward. This is usually a big incentive to avoid that epidural for lots of women!'
ELIDH PARSLOW AND LIZ NOONAN, BUMP CLASS MIDWIVES

44 Epidural

Whether or not you should have, might have, will have or won't have an epidural is one of the most talked about topics for expectant mothers. Some are adamant that labour without an epidural is a rite of passage on the road to motherhood, and others insist that they want one the moment they feel the first contraction. There are various scare stories about births with or without an epidural, and a lot of those stories have lost nothing (apart from their accuracy) in the telling. Make sure you know the facts and don't make any firm decisions until you are in labour.

 ## Commonly asked questions about epidurals

'What is an epidural?'
An epidural is an injection of local anaesthetic into the spinal fluid that takes away the pain of contractions completely.

'How commonly is it used?'
In England about 20 per cent of women have an epidural, which is lower than a lot of other western countries (in America it is almost 60 per cent).

'Who puts it in?'
It is always put in by an anaesthetist, a doctor who will have specifically trained in placing epidurals.

'How is it put in?
The anaesthetist will ask you to sit on the edge of the bed and to lean forward, curving your back as much as possible. They will inject local anaesthetic into the area where the epidural will be placed. This will sting a bit and is the only 'pain' you should experience during the whole procedure. You will feel a pushing sensation as a needle is used to access the space in the spine where the medication will be put. A thin soft tube is threaded through the needle and the needle is then removed. The needle is only used as a way to get the tube in the right place and does not stay in your back. The tube is taped on your back and a 'port' is attached to the end through which the medication can be given and 'topped up' when required. The anaesthetic given through the epidural numbs the body from the breasts down.

'Can it be put in while I am having a contraction?'

The anaesthetist is very used to putting epidurals in during labour and it is perfectly safe. It's important that you keep as still as possible so they'll try to put it in between contractions but, if while they're putting the epidural in, you feel a contraction coming, let them know.

'What is a "mobile epidural"?'

These days, epidurals are rather more sophisticated and it is now possible for you not to feel any pain but still be relatively mobile. Although you won't be quite as active as you would be without an epidural, you should be able to change positions on the bed and use gravity to assist the labour.

'How do I feel to "push" with an epidural?'

You won't have the natural urge to push with an epidural, so the midwife will monitor when you have a contraction and tell you when to push.

'Will it affect my baby?'

Because the medicine in an epidural is administered locally rather than into the blood, it does not get into the baby's body.

> *'I commonly come across patients who tell me that they want an epidural with the first contraction but then sail through labour without needing one. Of course there are others who make the decision not to have an epidural before labour starts and end up being disappointed when they have one. Whether or not you have an epidural is irrelevant; what is a shame is if having one makes a new mother disappointed. The birth of your baby is about so much more than the pain relief you needed and should be enjoyed however it happens.'* CHIARA

 ## The risks and benefits of an epidural
Benefits
It takes away the pain of labour, allowing an exhausted woman time to rest in preparation for the pushing.

Risks

- There may be side effects of the medication. Everyone responds differently but common side effects include a drop in blood pressure, causing you to feel light-headed or nauseous, and itching and feeling shivery.
- There is a chance of a 'dural puncture': when a membrane within the spine is accidentally punctured, which can lead to a headache. The headache can come on a day or two after the epidural. Typically you have the headache when standing or sitting but not when lying down. Treatment is straightforward so tell your doctor.
- Epidurals can slow contractions down and make the pushing stage of labour longer (although not by much – a recent study showed this to be only 13 minutes on average). The doctors may need to help speed up contractions again by giving you some oxytocin.
- The epidural might not work perfectly first time around. For example, it may only be effective on one side; in this case it would need to be resited.
- A catheter will need to be inserted into the bladder as the epidural's numbing affects the bladder. This is painless and usually uncomplicated but occasionally it can cause minor bladder problems for a day or two.

Common myths

'I should be worried about paralysis'

The risks of becoming paralysed as the result of an epidural are vanishingly rare. For paralysis to occur the spinal cord needs to be damaged. The spinal cord continues to about half way down your spine and below this are lots of nerves coming off it rather like a horse's tail, floating around in the spinal fluid. It is around these nerves, away from the spinal cord itself, that the epidural is inserted. While the needle may touch one of these 'tails' (often causing a feeling of electric shock in the legs), it can't damage the cord. This is a very simplistic explanation of an extremely complicated part of our anatomy but it's important that you understand why the terrifying risk of paralysis is so low. To put it into perspective, the chance of you having permanent damage as a result of an epidural in childbirth in the UK is less than 1 in 80,000.

'It might cause long-term back pain'

A recent review of lots of different studies concluded that there was no increased risk of this after an epidural.

'It will increase my chance of having a caesarean'

There have been studies that examine this theory and it is now widely considered that you are at no higher risk of having a caesarean if you have an epidural.

'It will increase my chance of having an assisted delivery (forceps or ventouse)'
Although there is a correlation between epidural and assisted delivery rates, once you've discounted the factors that are widely agreed to be the defining cause of needing an assisted delivery (such as a long latent phase, large baby or 'back to back' presentation), the risk is virtually insignificant. So basically, while a lot of women who have had epidurals might need an assisted delivery, it's not that the epidural caused this, but rather other factors.

'It is sometimes "too late" to have an epidural'
If you're pushing your baby out and it simply isn't coming and the doctors decide you need a caesarean section, they will put an epidural in. The only time when a midwife might suggest it is too late to have an epidural is if by the time you get an epidural in and working your baby will be born. It's not that they can't give you one, it's just that there's no point.

The main reason people choose not to have an epidural is that it medicalises the birth. Because of this you can't have an epidural in most midwife-led birth centres. With the epidural comes a drip in the vein, a catheter in the bladder and continuous monitoring of the baby and contractions. That said, there is no denying the huge relief that comes when the pain is suddenly gone, and 90 per cent of women who have had an epidural are pleased with the decision they have made.

45 Early labour *(the latent stage)*

As you approach 'term' you might well start to feel a little achy, uncomfortable and ready to have your baby. Do remember that term is from 37 weeks but first-time mothers are more likely to give birth closer to 41 weeks. You might have been having Braxton Hicks contractions from much earlier on in your pregnancy (see page 82). These are irregular, practice contractions that every pregnant woman will have. For some they are uncomfortable, but many don't even notice them.

Most women have what is called a 'show' up to 10 days before their labour starts. The cervix, which during your pregnancy has been tightly shut, has a mucus plug and, as your cervix starts to soften (or ripen), this plug is expelled. You will notice a clear jelly-like substance that is often tinged with streaks of blood. It might come out in one go, or it might come out over a few days.

 ## How does labour start?

Contractions

For most women the first sign that their labour is starting are contractions. These will probably start irregularly, and will be annoying but not very painful. Rather than dropping everything and texting your friends that your baby is coming, the best way to deal with early labour is to ignore it. Try as hard as you can to distract yourself; go for a walk, do some cooking or watch a film, but don't start timing every contraction. This is obviously a time to make sure your hospital bag is packed as it won't be long until your baby is born.

That said, the latent phase of labour can be exhaustingly long. Some women don't even notice it, but for others, often first-time mothers, this stage can last a day or two. Although it doesn't need to be your birth partner with you during this time, you should not be alone.

Waters breaking

For about 10 per cent of women the first sign of labour starting will be their waters breaking. Your baby is floating in a sac of amniotic fluid, rather like a water balloon. When the membranes rupture, the sac breaks and your waters (amniotic fluid) start leaking. Your waters can break at any point during your labour: from before contractions start to the moment your baby is born. Some babies are even born in their amniotic sacs; this unusual delivery is sometimes known as a mermaid birth or 'en caul' birth.

Waters breaking is not often like the depictions by Hollywood. For most women there will not be a huge gush of water flooding the area they're standing in; instead there will be a leak – more like if you've not quite made it to the loo in time.

Amniotic fluid can be confused with urine; it's sometimes straw-like or pinkish in colour, but it smells completely different. Extraordinarily it smells sweet and quite nice, a bit like fresh apple or pear drops – nothing like urine. So, if you're in doubt, give it a smell.

If your waters have broken, start wearing a sanitary pad immediately. Although you might not have to go into hospital, it's important to tell your midwife that your waters have broken.

> *'When you think labour might be imminent and your bodily fluids are changing, it's worth popping in a sanitary pad, so that if anything unusual comes out, you can show it to your midwife. Believe us, we will not be disgusted! We will always ask a lot about your bodily fluid's colour, consistency and smell. It may sound revolting but it's the best way for us to work out what is happening!' LIZ NOONAN AND ELIDH PARSLOW, BUMP CLASS MIDWIVES*

If you know that you are strep B-positive (see box below), you will need to tell your medical team this at this point. If you notice that the fluid from your waters is a slightly green or black colour you should call your midwife or the hospital. If there is any fresh bleeding this is not normal and you should go to the hospital immediately.

Group B Strep

Group B Streptococcus (GBS, or 'strep B') is a type of bacteria that can cause illness in people of all ages. Ten to 30 per cent of pregnant women carry this bacteria without having any symptoms. If you are carrying it at the time of delivery, there is a 50 per cent chance of passing it to your baby. If you do pass it on to your baby there is a 1–2 per cent chance of her developing a serious life threatening infection such as meningitis or septicemia. To treat strep B, intravenous antibiotics will be given to you in labour but that does not mean you cannot labour normally. You can still be upright and mobile and sometimes can even be in the water.

> **Group B Strep (continued)**
>
> In the UK the NHS do not screen for strep B but treat women with antibiotics if they have any signs in labour that they might be infected with it or if there is an increased risk of the mother transmitting infection to the baby.
>
> In the USA and much of Europe (as well as privately in the UK) pregnant women are screened at 37 weeks with a simple swab test. If it comes back positive then they are treated with antibiotics in labour to prevent the infection being transmitted to the baby. To be screened for strep B in the UK you need to arrange and pay for it privately.

What to do in early labour

For some this latent stage is the hardest bit, as mothers generally don't have the support of a midwife and it can take a long time, but there are lots of things you can do that will make dealing with this stage a lot easier:

- When there is still around 10 minutes between contractions, try to rest as much as possible. In between contractions you won't feel pain and it's important to use this time to rest. Try to find a position that is comfortable during a contraction, but that you can also rest in once the contraction stops. Often this will be kneeling, resting your arms on a chair or a Swiss ball, or using lots of pillows for support.
- When a contraction begins, breathe slowly and deeply, in through your nose and out through your mouth, keeping your breathing controlled and regular until the pain fades away.
- If you can't lie down, run a bath. If you're comfortable, stay there for a couple of hours but make sure there is someone within earshot to give you a hand when you need to get out.
- It's imperative that you keep yourself hydrated so have a bottle of water (ideally with a sports top) handy so you can sip water regularly. If you feel hungry eat what you feel like – most women like snacking on toast or fruit. You may feel nauseous or vomit at some point; that's normal.
- If you're feeling restless try to distract yourself – watch a film, bake a cake, do some cleaning!
- If you have a TENS machine, begin using it as soon as you feel you need a little bit of extra pain relief.
- If all else fails, go out for a long walk (not alone), and try to include hills. Keeping your pelvis moving helps move the baby down in the right direction.
- It's entirely normal to feel frustrated; try to think positively – each contraction is another step closer to your baby's arrival.

Kit for early labour

This stage of labour is exhausting so we suggest that you prepare a 'bag of tricks', each of which will help you a little bit through this stage. Try one thing and, if it's no longer helping, try the next one. Don't be afraid to try something again that hasn't worked before – often different things help at different stages and everything is worth a try.

- Paracetamol – take two tablets (1,000 mg) every 4–6 hours
- Go for a walk
- Make sure you're remembering your breathing techniques
- A selection of funny films
- Hot water bottle or heat pack
- Birthing ball – to lean on or bounce on
- Essential oils (such as lavender, clary sage)
- Have a warm bath or shower
- Wooden massage roller
- Plenty of pillows
- Your favourite music
- Isotonic drinks and snacks
- Visualisation/hypnotherapy audio tracks
- TENS machine
- Most importantly – REST!

Many Bump Class mothers say that they've found early labour the hardest part. It can go on for an annoyingly long time and all the while they feel like they are making so little progress. Although the cervix may have only dilated to 2 or 3 cm it's actually done a huge amount of work. From being tightly shut and long during your pregnancy, it's slowly shortened and softened and then started to dilate.

Throughout this stage you should be in regular contact with a midwife. If you have any doubts, call them and, if you feel that you would like to see someone, go into hospital. If they examine you and find that you are less than 3 cm dilated, they will encourage you to go home. This can be disheartening, but try to remember that the reason for this is that home is the best place for you at this stage.

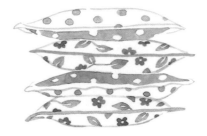

46 When to go *to hospital*

One of the things girls are most keen to know, and partners are most worried about, is when to go to hospital. You can go to hospital and you will be seen and assessed at any stage of your labour, and as a general rule you should go if you are at all worried or simply want reassurance.

> As soon as it feels like your labour might be starting you should be in contact with the hospital.

You should call the hospital at any time, but especially if:
- You are having contractions every 5 minutes
- You think your waters may have broken
- You are worried about your baby's movements
- You have any fresh bleeding

Always call them before you plan to leave for hospital.

Ideally the hospitals want you to come in when you're in active labour (so at least 4 cm dilated) and in most cases they would recommend that you go home if you're not yet at this stage. This said, if you really don't want to go home, then they will keep you in, on the antenatal ward. This is usually a cubicled ward with women at various stages of their pregnancy on it; it's not the ideal place to spend your latent phase, which is why the relaxed environment of home is usually encouraged.

How to know when you're in active labour
So we've established that the time to go to hospital is when you're in active labour, dilated to around 4 cm. But since you're unable to perform a vaginal examination on yourself (please don't even try this), how are you supposed to know when you reach this point?

The most important thing to remember is to trust your instinct and call or go into hospital if you feel you need to. Remember you don't need to go to hospital at exactly 4 cm; it's perfectly fine to arrive when you're 5, 6 or even 8 cm dilated.

Here are a few things that will indicate you're in active labour:

- Regular contractions every 3–5 minutes; regular means that there have been no intervals of longer than 3–5 minutes for the last couple of hours. Contrary to the latent phase – where you might have a series of regular contractions at 4-minute intervals combined with longer periods (say 20 minutes with no contractions) – contractions in active labour are usually so regular you can set your watch by them.
- Generally your contractions will be lasting around a minute.
- As opposed to the latent stage of labour, in active labour you won't usually be able to continue a conversation while you're having a contraction.

Reasons to go in to hospital before active labour

- If your waters break you should call but you won't necessarily need to go in. However, you do need to go in if your waters break and either you know you're strep B-positive (see pages 129–30), there is fresh bleeding (a small amount of pinkish liquor or a bloody show mixed in is normal) or if the waters are discoloured (greeny brown rather than straw-coloured) or offensive smelling.
- It's not normal to have a fever in labour. If you suspect you might, take your temperature, and, if you do, go in to hospital.
- Your baby should be moving normally during labour; if you have any concerns that it's not, go in.

We explain the importance of your birth environment on page 121; labour which has often been progressing nicely at home, may slow down as soon as the mother reaches hospital. It's worth making every effort to make the transfer from home to hospital as smooth and relaxed as possible and hopefully your labour will then proceed more quickly.

47 Active *labour*

This stage of labour is sometimes referred to as 'the first stage of labour', which we think is a little unfair; it suggests that the often long and uncomfortable latent stage is insignificant or not 'proper' labour. Actually for many, it's the hardest part and it's important to keep your spirits up. For this reason, we prefer to refer to this next stage of labour as 'active labour' – which reflects the reality much more accurately!

'Active labour' is when:
- The cervix dilates from 4 cm to 10 cm – wide enough for the baby to be born.
- Contractions are strong and regular with no prolonged rest periods. Generally they come 3–5 minutes apart and last for 1–2 minutes. Please understand that this is by no means a given; it varies from woman to woman.
- By this stage, you will be going to or be at hospital or, if you're giving birth at home, a midwife will be supporting you.

> *'I've seen all sorts of women behaving very differently during contractions: some keep completely silent and withdraw into themselves; others become quite animalistic and make loud, often bizarre noises, which helps them through the contractions. Whatever method you find is helping, it is important to try to remain relaxed, calm and in control. Midwives agree that the more relaxed the woman, the faster the labour progresses, which is why many mothers have quick labours at home. However, at the time of writing, studies have shown that, for first-time mothers, the safest place to deliver the baby is in hospital or a birth centre attached to a hospital.' CHIARA*

 ## What happens in active labour?
When you get into hospital you will be taken to an assessment area where they perform the usual antenatal checks on both the mother and baby. You will also be offered a vaginal examination (VE): the only way of knowing for sure how dilated you are. This is when a midwife or doctor performs an internal examination to feel the cervix, estimating with their fingers the dilation of the cervix. It sounds hideous but in reality it is not too bad; it takes a matter of minutes and, although

not particularly pleasant, most women agree that it is no worse than having a smear test (and generally quicker).

'Do I have to have a VE?'

Q&A

You would never be forced to have one, but once labour has started, most women want to know how far along they are. Having said that, if it is clear to the midwives that you are progressing nicely with regular strong contractions and there are no concerns about the baby, then it is not always necessary to have an examination. Some women will deliver their baby never having had a VE. The important thing is not to be scared of it. No one can predict whether or not you will need examining, although the likelihood is that you will, so keep an open mind.

Once they have established that you're in active labour, you will be given your own room and a dedicated midwife, who will support you through your labour. Do bear in mind that they usually work on 12-hour shifts, so depending on the timing and duration of your labour, you may have more than one midwife.

Throughout active labour the midwife will listen to the baby's heart rate regularly, and, if there are any medical interventions or concerns about the baby or how the labour is progressing, you may be continuously monitored with a machine strapped to your abdomen listening to the heartbeat and checking the contractions.

If they haven't done so already, your waters may break at any time during this stage; this is a good sign that labour is progressing.

Try to keep as mobile and active as possible and continue to change positions. If a position has not worked for you earlier on in labour, try it again later. There are many different positions that work brilliantly and some women will find some better than others. Midwives are great at suggesting different positions that will help you with the intensity of contractions and get the baby into a good position for delivery. Take advantage of your midwife's knowledge and experience.

Remember to balance being mobile with having periods of rest between your contractions. This is particularly important if your labour is going on slightly longer.

Once in active labour, your options for pain relief are broadened but will include techniques and aids that you may have been using up to this point, such as:

- Breathing
- Hypnotherapy and visualisation
- Keeping upright and mobile
- Massage
- TENS machine
- Paracetamol

There are also a number of pain-relief options that are usually only recommended once you're in active labour:

- Birth pool
- Gas and air
- Pethidine
- Epidural

See page 118 for further information on the various forms of pain relief.

'Will I be able to eat and drink in active labour?'
If you have not had an epidural, you can eat and drink as you like and you will probably find that small high-energy snacks and drinks are what you will feel like.

Q&A

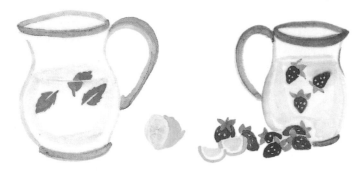

The trials of transition

Transition is when the cervix approaches 10 cm at the end of the active stage of labour. It's probably the most difficult, but thankfully one of the shortest, parts of labour. It is common for women to feel very out of control at this stage. You will feel increasing amounts of pressure in your bottom and will probably feel like giving up, packing your bags and going home. Unfortunately, labour won't stop if you do! Many women also become quite different in personality during this stage, even becoming rude and aggressive to whomever is around – midwives, husbands and mothers all take the hit! Your partner will probably be mortified but, rather than taking offence, the medical team will be delighted, as this is a good sign that your labour is progressing nicely and your baby's arrival is imminent.

This is often the time when a woman who has coped beautifully in labour using natural techniques, suddenly feels she needs an epidural as she can no longer cope without one. Rather than her needing an epidural, this is the hormonal change of transition talking and so the midwives will often support her through this period, encouraging her to continue as she has, in the knowledge that, rather like the sprint to the finish line, if she has got this far, the worst is over.

Transition is thankfully short-lived, but it's worth anticipating it and warning your birth partner that hormonal changes may temporarily change your behaviour.

Some things Bump Class girls have shouted during transition*:
- 'I wish I'd never married you.'
- 'I've changed my mind, I'm not having this baby.'
- 'This is the biggest mistake of my life.'
- (To the obstetrician) 'And by the way that's the most disgusting tie I've ever seen.'
- ... and quite a few more that are unprintable ...

*All marriages survived ... and most mothers have gone on to have second children.

48 Pushing and the *delivery of the placenta*

The next stage of labour is when the cervix is fully dilated and you are pushing your baby out. Women who haven't had an epidural will feel an overwhelming urge to push with every contraction. Try not to be frightened. Listen to your body and go with it. If you do have an epidural you may still feel pressure but your midwife will need to guide you as to when and how to push.

How to push your baby out

- If you can, keep mobile and follow your midwife's directions using different positions. At this stage you want gravity on your side so arguably lying on your back to deliver your baby is counterproductive. Depending on the circumstances it's not always possible to be upright, but it's worth trying if you can. Even if you have an epidural in, many women find that kneeling, squatting, being on all fours or even standing works for them. You need to push with your contractions and, rather than just getting through them, work with them to help your baby be born.
- Push long and hard into your bottom. The feeling when pushing should be the same as if you were very constipated and trying to open your bowels.
- Pushing is tiring. Use your energy only for pushing and rest between contractions.
- Some women make a lot of noise while pushing. Rather than wasting energy making noise, try to use every ounce of your energy for pushing. Bringing your head forward with your chin on your chest can help you to focus this energy really efficiently.

★ Getting around 'the U-bend'

As the baby's head descends through the birth canal, it needs to pass under your pubic bone, which is a bit like going through a U-bend. As a result you will feel the baby's head rocking back and forth. It can feel like two steps forward, one step back. As frustrating as this may feel, it is actually really important as it helps to stretch the tissues slowly, which prevents tearing.

Once the baby's head has passed the 'bend', you will no longer feel the rocking and instead you will feel a stretching sensation as the baby's head is 'crowning', or being born. At this point the midwife will ask you to stop pushing and 'pant' instead. It's quite common to feel an urge to just push the baby's head out and get it over with, but this is the time, almost more than any other, to focus on exactly what your midwife is telling you to do. You should follow their instructions exactly as they are trying to ensure that your baby's head is born slowly, gently stretching the tissues and minimising the risk of tearing.

In the vast majority of cases, delivering the head is the hard part. The body usually comes very easily in the next one or two contractions. Remember though that there are usually a few minutes between contractions even at this stage, so you may find that your baby's head is born and there is a bit of a wait before the rest of her arrives. Don't worry, this is perfectly normal. When the next contraction comes, you will need to push strongly again to deliver the body and then your baby is born!

Something to warn your partner about

Let's face it, the idea of having a few minutes where your baby's head is poking out of your vagina while you wait for the rest of her to be born can be … unnerving. Some fathers will be curious to take a first look at their baby. It's worth warning them that babies are not usually crying at this point and the head might well look a bit blue, which is fine. At this stage your baby is still getting all she needs from the placenta and very often will not take her first breath until she's been delivered. Often fathers expecting to meet their rosy-cheeked cherubs have a bit of a shock!

 ## What happens when your baby is born

If all is well your midwife will deliver your baby straight onto your chest for your first cuddle and loosely cover her with a towel. This is a wonderful moment that no mother ever forgets and it gives you the chance to have your first skin-to-skin cuddle and feed (see page 156 for more on this). Newborn babies are a bit mucky, often covered with a bit of their mother's blood and the greasy vernix that has protected their skin in the amniotic fluid. Although before birth this sounds a little off-putting, most mothers are so delighted to finally have their baby in their arms that they don't even notice. If, however, you'd rather your baby is quickly wiped down and wrapped up before being given to you, no one will think any less of you as a mother. The important thing is that you enjoy the experience.

Vitamin K injection

It is recommended that babies have vitamin K, by injection, in the first few hours of life to prevent the development of an early bleeding tendency known as 'haemorrhagic disease of the newborn'. Although rare, this disease is entirely preventable with very safe treatment. (If no baby was given vitamin K at birth, 17 babies in 1,000 would contract the disease with a high mortality rate.)

The injection is a once-only dose that provides protection against haemorrhage in the first few weeks of life. Vitamin K can also be given orally, but this is then three doses – at birth, one week and one month of age. This may not provide as much protection to your baby as we cannot be sure how much the baby receives. No side effects have been found with vitamin K by injection or orally.

> *'I would always recommend that you opt for the vitamin K injection. If it's given orally it's given to you to take home and give at one week and one month – and it's another thing to remember to do. I've also tasted it and it's bitter and disgusting. Babies' first taste is usually sweet-tasting colostrum rather than this bitter medicine, so I'd argue that it's kinder on your baby to give her a quick injection (which after being pushed through the birth canal will not be a big deal). The other thing to bear in mind is that babies who are given the vitamin K orally are generally given six times the amount as the injection because it's difficult to work out what they actually swallow rather than spit out.'*
> LIZ NOONAN, BUMP CLASS MIDWIFE

 ## The dreaded question of tearing or being cut 'down there'

This is most first-time mothers' biggest fear. Quite tellingly, sleep deprivation after the baby is born is what most second-time mothers fear the most! The one thing that most women confirm after they've become mothers is that, if it happens, it's not as bad as it sounds and generally heals very well.

As the baby is crowning, your perineum has to stretch significantly and it's not uncommon for there to be a small tear. We don't mean a gaping wound – it's more like a small nick which often doesn't even require any stitches and heals very well on its own. Sometimes when tears are more substantial, they do need stitches.

Sometimes tears are more substantial, and this is what doing an episiotomy is trying to prevent. An episiotomy is a small, controlled cut that gives more space for the baby's head to come out. It is not standard practice to have an episiotomy. The doctor or midwife will make the decision at the moment of birth. It is usually only

'Why do some people choose not to have the oxytocin injection?'
Some people prefer simply not to have any medical intervention in
their labour, regardless of whether there are any known negative effects
on the mother or baby. Anyone choosing not to have this injection should be
aware of the fact that the risk of heavy bleeding is increased, and this, in rare
circumstances, can lead to women requiring a blood transfusion. If you've had any
medical intervention at all (assisted delivery or epidural), you will need to have the
injection and it would be considered irresponsible to refuse; it is strongly advised
that you have this injection.

'Will my baby cry immediately?'
It is quite common for it to take a few moments for your baby to start breathing on
her own and crying after birth but this can seem like an eternity. Babies can look
a little blue and floppy immediately after birth and the midwife will rub her down
vigorously to stimulate her breathing. There are amazing physiological changes
going on in your baby's body at the moment of birth. The blood vessels to and
from the lungs are used for the first time as she takes the first breaths. The hole in
the heart that has been bypassing the lungs closes as she starts breathing. It is not
surprising that this sometimes takes a little time, so try not to worry.

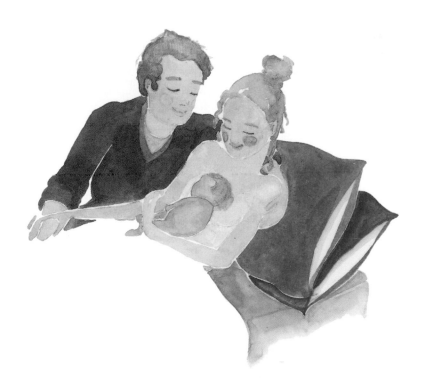

done if it looks like otherwise there may be a nasty tear, which may go all the way down into the muscles that control your bladder and bowel, sometimes through to the rectum. An episiotomy, even though it sounds brutal, is preferable to this.

An episiotomy may be done by a doctor or a midwife, and this or any larger tear would be stitched once the baby has been born and the placenta delivered. You will be given local anaesthetic (if you don't have an epidural) and this should not be at all painful. If it is, let them know and they will give you more anaesthetic. Once in, the stitches are dissolvable and do not need to be removed.

Most women who have had an episiotomy have found it was in no way as bad as they had imagined beforehand. The vaginal tissue heals particularly well and remarkably quickly, and most people barely give their stitches a second thought afterwards.

'What if I do a poo in labour?'

Q&A

This is a question we get asked on every Bump Class. When one girl finally plucks up the courage to ask the question that every girl is thinking about there is a palpable collective sigh, as it's generally something every pregnant person worries about. The reality is that doing what is usually a very small poo in labour is very common but the good news is that, if it does happen, you're probably not going to realise it's happened. As the baby passes down the birth canal it puts pressure on the rectum so every woman will feel like they are doing a poo, even if that's not the case. The midwives are constantly changing the disposable pads at your bottom end – amniotic fluid is persistently leaking – and so if a little poo comes out, they quickly wrap it away in the pad and get rid of it. It is very unlikely that either you or your birth partner will be aware it has happened and the midwife is certainly not going to draw attention to it! It's really important we talk about this because if you're afraid of doing a poo as you're pushing, you'll be afraid to push. And you really need to push, very hard, without any restraint.

Interestingly, women are so scared about this before labour, but we speak to every girl after they've given birth and not one, in the history of The Bump Class, has ever mentioned whether or not they did a poo. This is not because they're embarrassed to tell us, but because it is of no consequence.

The delivery of the placenta

The final stage of labour is the delivery of the placenta and, for most women, this stage will all but pass them by. They are normally too busy admiring their perfect baby for the first time to notice much.

All women are recommended to have an injection of oxytocin to aid this stage (see page 141). This assists the separation of the placenta from the lining of the uterus and helps the uterus contract, thereby reducing the risk of having heavy bleeding. With the injection, the placenta comes out within about 15 minutes of the birth with minimal effort. If you choose not to have the injection, this stage will take about an hour and you will need to push the placenta out. It is widely agreed that there are no significant risks associated with the injection and any potential risks are greatly outweighed by the benefits. By the time you have the injection, the umbilical cord will have been cut so the baby cannot be affected.

Q&A

'Are there any benefits to eating my placenta?'

In the last couple of decades some people have suggested that there might be some benefits for the mother to eat her placenta. There are companies that will dry the placenta and make it into pills that the mother can easily eat. Some people just fry up the fresh placenta or make it into a spaghetti bolognese … They argue that eating it can ward off postnatal depression and boost milk supply, plus since it's packed with nutrients, vitamins and iron, it can help women recover postnatally. While it's true that the placenta contains lots of potentially beneficial nutrients and hormones, there is no evidence to suggest that well-nourished mothers can gain any benefit from eating their placenta that cannot be gained elsewhere.

The other argument is that many mammals eat their placenta, and since we're 'just mammals' this is something we should also do. However, we've also evolved and there are plenty of things that mammals do that we simply don't – like eating excrement and eating our children to preserve our alpha status. It's thought that the reason vulnerable mammals do eat their placentas is to destroy the evidence of a recent birth from predators. That said, there's probably no harm in eating your placenta, so if it's something you feel very strongly that you'd like to do just make sure you go about it in a sensible fashion and seek appropriate advice.

49 Assisted *delivery*

Every woman hopes to have her baby with as little medical intervention as possible, but there are some circumstances where the medical team looking after you may feel that it is safer for you and your baby if they help a bit. It is impossible to predict how your labour will progress and it is therefore important to understand all the different courses it can take. If you are prepared for all eventualities and aware of the terminology used, then you are more likely to remain confident and in control whatever happens.

> *'I advise my patients that, rather than feeling disappointed that they have needed some intervention, they should be thankful that they were able to deliver their babies somewhere where that expert help was readily available. Had it not been, the outcome may have been different. As a doctor, I can assure you that we would be delighted if we never had to be involved in childbirth; in an ideal world all births would be straightforward and a midwife is the ideal person to deal with a straightforward birth. However, the reality is that one in eight women have complications and require a doctor's input for both their and their baby's well-being.' CHIARA*

Any decision to intervene is not taken lightly and that decision will only be made if it is felt that it really is necessary. Essentially an assisted delivery is simply the medical team becoming involved in assisting the baby's delivery in the pushing stage, commonly if the baby needs a little help getting around that 'U-bend'.

Common reasons for assisting are if:
- There is a prolonged pushing stage of labour – if you've been pushing for a long time
- The baby is in an awkward position
- There are concerns about the baby's heart rate or signs of fetal distress
- There is a medical reason for her not to push for too hard or for too long
- The mother is too exhausted to push effectively

How your baby is monitored

During your labour your baby's heart rate will be monitored, either intermittently using a Doppler machine, or continuously. If there are any concerns, the doctor or midwife is sometimes able to take a small sample of the baby's blood, which can be analysed by a machine to give a more accurate idea of how she is doing. This is done by making a small scratch on her head during a vaginal examination. It doesn't hurt the baby and the scratch heals very quickly once she is born.

What might be used?

The two instruments generally used to aid labour are forceps or suction devices (sometimes known as ventouse).

- Forceps are smooth metal instruments that look like large spoons or tongs. They lock into place so you don't need to worry that they are going to squash your baby's head.
- A ventouse is a small round cup that attaches to the back of the head by creating a vacuum.

Both of these instruments can be used to guide the baby out, rotate her head and provide traction for the obstetrician to help deliver. The doctor can use these to gently guide the baby out in conjunction with the mother's pushing. It is a team effort.

The choice of instrument will depend on the position of the baby and the preference of the doctor. There is not one method that is 'better' than the other, and you should not have a preference over which method the doctor uses. Instead rest assured that the only consideration is what is best for you and your baby in your situation.

It is often done in an operating theatre, mainly because, in the unlikely event that it is unsuccessful, you are in the right place for them to do a caesarean quickly. In order to give your baby as much space as possible, your legs will need to be put into supports. A paediatrician may be present to check your baby once it is born.

If all is well, your baby can be delivered onto your chest, and your birthing partner may still be able to cut the cord if they want to. You may notice that the forceps leave small marks on the baby's face and that the ventouse leaves a bruise on the head, but these will disappear very quickly.

Although not always the case, it may be necessary to have an episiotomy with an assisted delivery. This is not as bad as it sounds – see page 140.

50 Caesarean *section*

'There is good evidence to suggest that, for uncomplicated pregnancies, the safest way to give birth is vaginally, and I would not advocate a caesarean section without a good medical reason. It is certainly not the easy option. However, sometimes the safest way to deliver your baby is by caesarean, and sometimes it is the only safe way.' CHIARA

There are two types of caesarean sections: elective and emergency.

- An elective caesarean is when the decision to have a caesarean has been made before labour starts. Although the name implies that you're making the choice, it's often for medical reasons, such as if the baby is breech or there is a low-lying placenta. It does not necessarily mean that the mother is 'too posh to push'.
- An emergency caesarean is when the decision is made once labour has started. Although the medics will be keen not to waste time, this does not necessarily mean the drama of flashing blue lights; often the experience is one of relative calm and the staff should have time to explain why this should happen.

Why you might need a caesarean

There are lots of reasons your doctor may advise a caesarean, either before or during labour. The most common reasons for an elective caesarean are:

- Breech position
- Twins
- Multiple/previous caesarean section(s)
- Placenta praevia (see page 73)

The most common reasons for emergency caesarean are:

- Fetal distress
- Failure to progress (cervix not dilating as it should)
- Bleeding in labour

This is by no means an exhaustive list, and, if your doctors are recommending that you have one, it's crucial to listen carefully why this is. Make sure that you understand and are involved in the decision-making. Even in an emergency, the doctors should take the time to explain the decision to you and make sure that you are happy with it. You will never be forced to do anything that you are unhappy with. Remember the best result for the medical team is also for you to have an uncomplicated vaginal delivery and they do have your and your baby's best interests at heart. If you are unsure about decisions being made, ask to speak to the consultant.

Why it is not the 'easy option'

Although for some women the birth itself seems easier with less effort involved on their part, having a caesarean is not the easy option. Major abdominal surgery carries relatively significant risks of complications. As with any surgery, there are risks of bleeding and infection. There are also the separate risks of having an epidural or potentially a general anaesthetic. In addition, there is no doubt that the first few weeks after the birth is much harder if you have had a caesarean, particularly if you have an older child at home. You have to stay in hospital longer after the birth and the overall recovery time is longer.

Studies have also shown that some childhood illnesses may be linked to their mother having had a caesarean. This is clearly something you need to be aware of, especially if you are considering having a caesarean without good medical reason.

For the vast majority of women the decision to have a caesarean is out of their hands. The doctors advise a caesarean because the risk of natural birth in that individual scenario is thought to outweigh the risk of the caesarean.

> 'I had twins by caesarean section a year after my older daughter was born naturally. The babies had reflux and it was intense having three children under two at home. Had I been able to have a natural delivery, these first weeks would have been so much easier. Recovering from a major operation was just another difficult thing at an already challenging time. That said, the decision was made in my and my boys' best interests, and ultimately the fact that we're all healthy is something I'm grateful for.' ALICE, THE BUMP CLASS

What is it like to have a caesarean section?

It is usually a relaxed environment. The radio will be playing or you can choose music that you want. The anaesthetist will be chatting to you and will be with you all the time.

There are often a surprising amount of people in the room during a caesarean. This is always something we warn The Bump Class about so they don't worry that the team might be

Dear Marina and Chiara,

I just wanted to let you know that my baby was born by caesarean yesterday late afternoon after a gruelling two-and-a-half days of labour!

I was devastated to find out I'd need a caesarean after so many hours of labour, but you were absolutely correct: it is no less magical ... an emergency caesarean was the last thing on my mind, seeing as I was booked into the birth centre (!), so I am truly grateful that you gave it the time of day during our classes as it made the experience far less harrowing.

Selma

especially worried in their situation. In a straightforward elective caesarean there might well be up to 10 people in the room, and it's standard to have a paediatric team there in an emergency caesarean, increasing that number. They all have a role and a lot of those roles are precautionary. Understandably they don't like to take risks – which is a good thing!

Unless there is an unusual situation, you will be awake during the surgery. Before surgery starts you will have an intravenous line inserted and the epidural will be placed in the operating theatre. You will have a catheter inserted and the area around the incision will be shaved. You will be on a firm narrow bed under the operating light. You may feel like you are going to fall off the bed. Don't worry, you won't; you're strapped on!

A screen will be put up between your head and lower body so that you can't see any of the operation. There are lots of machines around you – they are standard. Try to ignore these. You are usually allowed one person with you in the operating theatre. They will be asked to wear surgical scrubs and will sit on a stool next to your head. The anaesthetist will be with you and can answer any questions.

A caesarean is always done by a doctor. They will make a small incision just above your pubic bone, trying to keep this as small as possible. Your muscles will then be pulled aside (not cut, as so many women believe) and another incision will be made in your uterus. Regardless of whether your waters have broken, there will still be amniotic fluid around your baby and they'll use a suction machine, similar to what the dentist uses, to remove the water. This is good to know as, when you hear this noise, you know your baby is about to be born. As this happens, you will feel a tugging or pulling sensation as well as a lot of pressure on your tummy, where one of the surgeons is pushing your baby from behind to help her out. You may be asked if you want the screen lowering a bit so that you can see the baby just after she is born. Your baby is usually out within 15 minutes of starting the operation. The rest of the operation can take another 40 minutes or so, but it will pass very quickly as you will be looking at your baby for the first time!

Your baby will usually be quickly checked by the midwife or paediatrician before being given to you or your partner to hold (usually wrapped in blankets) but you can have skin-to-skin contact if you want to. Once the operation is finished you will transfer from the operating theatre to the recovery room, where you will be for about an hour for monitoring, assuming all is well. This is a good time for skin-to-skin contact and breastfeeding, which you should try to do as soon as you can (see page 156).

Once the doctors are happy that all is well and you are stable, you will be moved to a postnatal room. The epidural will wear off over the next few hours and you will slowly be allowed to eat and drink. Most women stay in hospital for two or three nights. The midwives will encourage you to get up and about as soon as possible. This will feel very sore at first but it gets better very quickly and mobilising will speed up your recovery.

Most girls on The Bump Class are hoping and preparing for a natural birth. However, it's crucial to spend time talking about what it's actually like to have a caesarean in case it's something you have to face.

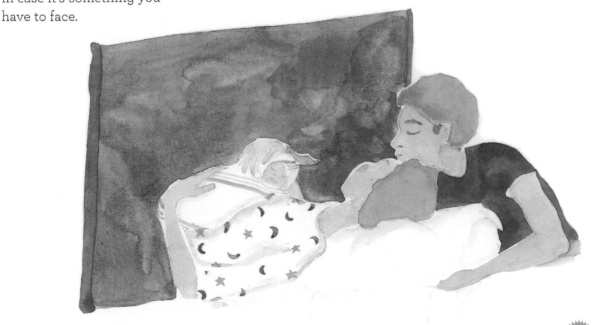

51 Becoming a father:
Your role during labour

You may not be the one actually giving birth, but you nevertheless have a crucial role. We often liken labour to a marathon; if this is the marathon of your partner's life, imagine that you're her pacer. You need to make sure she's prepared and has the tools to help her, and once those contractions start you should encourage her, help her conserve her strength and energy and, above all, keep positive.

 ### Early labour
This is when you will probably be at home, so arguably the part where she needs you most.

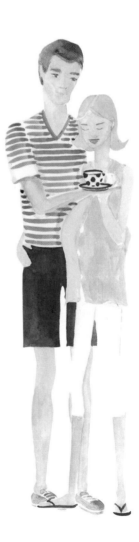

- Be aware of what will be happening physiologically and how she will feel; read pages 128–31.
- Distract her; when contractions start, make a plan to go for a walk, go shopping or watch a funny film. If it happens to be night-time, encourage her to sleep in between the contractions. She should still have 10 minutes or so in between contractions, and if she can doze then it will help her hugely. Help her find a position in which she's as comfortable as possible during a contraction but in which she can rest in between them. This will often be upright, leaning on something or propped up with lots of cushions.
- Make sure she's breathing properly through the contractions (see page 119).
- Give her paracetamol to take every 4–6 hours. Set an alarm to make sure she takes them regularly, as this is when they are most effective.
- Get her into the bath; water is great for pain relief. Don't leave her alone – the water will need constant topping up and she might need help shifting position. Make sure everywhere she feels pain is covered in water. Focusing a hand shower on these parts really helps.

- Massage her lower back. A lot of women find that hard massage at the base of the spine is really helpful but others hate being touched – be led by her.
- If you have a TENS machine, get it out and work out how to use it. It has clear instructions.
- If she's coping well by herself, try to have some rest yourself, particularly if it's night-time. You will be much more helpful to her if you're not exhausted.
- Make sure her hospital bags are packed and ready to go and that you've got her medical notes to bring to the hospital.
- Have a look at the 'bag of tricks' (page 131) and, when she feels that one thing is no longer working, be ready to suggest the next and convince her that it will help.

 ## When to go into hospital

- Try not to go in too early but stay in regular contact with the hospital. Try to speak to the same person if you can – they will have a better overview of her labour as a whole.
- Generally speaking, the time to go into hospital is when the contractions are coming regularly, every 3–5 minutes apart, and she's unable to continue a conversation while the contraction is at its peak.
- Listen to your partner – if she wants to go into hospital, go in.
- Call the hospital if her waters break – they might not need you to go in immediately, but it's something they need to know.
- If there's any fresh blood at any time, go into hospital urgently.
- Read page 132, which covers this in detail.

When you get to hospital or the birth centre they will examine your partner – they'll check the baby's heartbeat, her blood pressure and they will also offer her a vaginal examination to see how dilated she is. This is the only way they can accurately ascertain how established her labour is. It's discreet and quick, although sometimes uncomfortable. During the examination, you will be more than welcome to stay with her if you both want.

If they establish that she is less than 4 cm dilated, you will be encouraged to go home. This can be demoralising for an exhausted woman, but home really is the best place for women in this stage of labour. Try to be upbeat and positive and encourage her to do the same.

The importance of positivity

Keep in mind that you are your partner's pacer. You need to be organised, but also keep her morale up. When she thinks she can't do it, you're the one persuading her that she can. The latent stage is a time when women often feel frustrated and demoralised. If they've established that she's only 2 cm dilated, she might understandably feel despondent. Even if you feel the same way, it's your job to eke every ounce of positivity from the situation to boost her spirits and give her the energy to keep on going.

Positive ways to interpret a 'disappointing' vaginal examination

- 'Don't be demoralised; think of all the work your body has done to get your cervix to 2 cm already.'
- 'It's good that this process is slow because it allows time for the tissues to stretch.'
- 'The latent stage is often the hardest stage. If it's long, it doesn't mean the rest of your labour will be long too; many women go on to have a quick active and pushing stage.'
- 'It's not going to be long until we meet our baby, which will be the best reward in world.'
- Get her to embrace each contraction rather than fear it, and remind her that 'every contraction is one less contraction to meeting our baby.'

A few of the worst things you could possibly say

- 'Seriously, all this time, and only 2 cm?'
- 'How long is this going to go on for?'
- 'I'm so tired.'

If she feels that she really can't go home, she can always stay in hospital, although this will probably be on the antenatal ward, which is far less comfortable than being at home, and you might not be able to stay with her.

Active labour

If your partner is 4 cm or more dilated, they will admit you both into your own room on the labour ward and a midwife will be assigned to you. This person (shift depending) will be with you throughout your labour to the birth of your baby.

Midwives are generally amazing people. Their job elicits great joy and they're brilliant at it and excellent at communicating with women in labour. Do try to make an effort with your midwife, but if for any reason she's struggling to bond or you feel that your partner is being inadequately supported, politely ask the midwife in charge of the ward if there's any chance of changing.

Once women are in established labour, they often feel empowered by the fact that things are moving along. They also have a new centre of support in the midwife, who will really assist them in labour. Your partner will be encouraged to use the water or gas and air and a variety of things that help women in labour. If she wants, she can also have an epidural at this stage. It's worth you becoming familiar with the various methods of pain relief, both natural and medical; have a look at page 118–23 for an overview of the pain-relief options. For those women who choose to have an epidural, the pain stops entirely and the rest of this stage will be more of a waiting game. Do use this time to get some sleep and encourage your partner to rest as well.

If she chooses not to have an epidural, she will need your support much more. *Beware of the transitional stage.* You might have heard about the stage when women who have been labouring really well suddenly think they can no longer cope and often try to pack their bags and leave the hospital. Physiologically, it's the final part of the active stage of labour, when a woman is transitioning into the pushing stage. A huge wave of adrenaline is released and often women turn into complete monsters. It's relatively short-lived but it's crucial that partners are prepared for this, as the last thing she needs is for you to take offence at something she says.

Transition is something that fathers need to be prepared for so read 'The trials of transition' on page 137.

 ## The pushing stage
The joy of transition is that you're on the home straight of labour. The pushing stage usually lasts an hour or two, and at the end you'll have something that was worth waiting for. During the pushing stage it's crucial that she listens to and follows the instructions of the midwife, and you might need to help the midwife here. Being a couple, you already have an understanding and trust, and it's often easier for someone who knows her to communicate these important instructions.

Your baby's head will be born and the rest of the body will follow in the next couple of contractions. Some fathers are curious to see the head born but it's something you need to have thought about beforehand. If you do have a look, bear in mind that the baby might look quite blue and lifeless – she's not breathing on her own yet, as her oxygen is coming from the placenta. For some this is disturbing and for others it's magical. If it's not for you, stay up at the head end. Deciding you don't want to watch your baby being born will not have any bearing on your abilities as a father.

We insist on preparing fathers for what their babies might look like – so do have a good read of page 139. Most expectant fathers' only experience of childbirth comes from Hollywood, which is entirely unrealistic.

After a straightforward birth your baby will be delivered straight onto her mother's chest. As important as this 'skin to skin' time is emotionally for mother and baby, it seems to have some physical benefits too. Studies have shown that the body heat and sound of the heartbeat calm babies down after the shock of being born. Interestingly, it doesn't matter who is holding him; the baby will still benefit and we encourage all fathers to have some skin-to-skin time with their babies. After a caesarean mothers often find it difficult to have skin-to-skin time so take this opportunity; she'll be more comfortable holding her child when she's out of theatre, in recovery.

> ## An emotional rollercoaster for partners too
> Mothers often say that just after the birth they're predominantly relieved, exhausted and ready for a cup of tea, with the emotion hitting a little later. Fathers on the other hand are often surprised at how emotional they are, even if they're not normally 'cryers'. Whatever you feel, enjoy the moment and don't feel embarrassed by your emotions. It's a moment that you will remember for ever.

Delivery of the placenta
The final stage of labour, the delivery of the placenta, will not concern you too much. We advise that if you're at all squeamish, don't watch. It's probably the goriest part of labour and you will have your amazing baby to watch instead!

Medical interventions in labour
Most couples hope for a straightforward birth but it's important to understand what would happen if any medical intervention is needed. This may be an assisted delivery, where the doctors would 'assist' the baby's birth using forceps or suction

device, or a caesarean section. We talk these in more detail on pages 145 and 146. As no one can predict the kind of birth they will have, we really recommend that you read these pages. If you are prepared and you know what the doctors are doing and why, you'll feel more in control and therefore less anxious. Try to be positive about it and thankful that this expert help is available if it's needed; it will obviously only be done if it's thought to be in your partner and baby's best interests.

 ## The postnatal ward

After your baby is safely delivered, as long as all is well, mother and baby will be transferred to the postnatal ward. Having had one-to-one care in a private room, the postnatal ward can be a little bit of a shock, but fathers can make this more comfortable.

- Try to spend as much time with your partner in the postnatal ward as you can – just being an extra pair of hands will be a huge help.
- Hospital food is rarely good and your partner will probably feel very hungry after labour, so do bring some food in for her. Don't guess what you think she'd like – ask her. Having been through labour, postnatal women are often craving something specific.
- Before she's discharged from hospital, make sure she has enough painkillers. Women often say that they are in more pain at home than they were at hospital – probably because they are being more active – so make sure you have plenty of painkillers.
- If she needs them, make sure she takes them regularly; women recover better if they are pain-free so don't let her be a martyr.
- The chances are that you'll have the opportunity to go home before your partner and baby return; if you do, tidy the house and clean up a little. Things might be a little messy if she has laboured there, and coming home to a tidy, homely house (fresh flowers are a winner) will make a huge difference.
- Try to fill the fridge with her favourite food that is easy to prepare; breastfeeding women are extraordinarily hungry so think about pre-cooked meals and nutritious snacks.

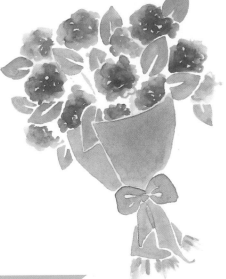

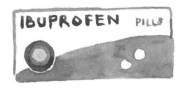

52 The *first feed*

From the moment your baby is born and placed on your chest, her instinct will be to find a nipple and start feeding. Amazingly, in spite of not even being able to hold up their heads, most babies are capable of wriggling up their mother's chest until they can find the nipple. Instead of placing your baby on the breast, do see if she can do this – it's an amazing thing to watch.

From as early as 20 weeks mothers may be producing colostrum, a sweet nectar-like substance that precedes breast milk and contains an incredible host of nutrients and antibodies that will give your baby the very best start to life. At birth your baby's stomach is approximately the size of a marble so you only produce tiny amounts of colostrum.

Try to feed your baby as soon as you can. As long as there are no major concerns for you or your baby, this can be pretty much straightaway if you have had a natural birth. For some mothers this might even be before the placenta has been delivered. Feeding means your baby is skin to skin, and this will ease the shock of her arrival into the world.

'As tough as my labour was, the moment they placed my daughter on my chest, none of it mattered.' SOPHIA, THE BUMP CLASS

Ideally the baby needs to get as much of the breast tissue in her mouth as possible. It's worth reading a little on breastfeeding before you go into labour so you're aware of what you're encouraging the baby to do. Getting a good latch early on will prevent you from getting sore nipples.

As soon as your baby has latched on and is sucking, you might well feel quite intense abdominal cramping. As painful as this can be, it's brilliant because it's your uterus contracting. Usually the size of a fist, your uterus has grown over your pregnancy to the size of a watermelon in order to accommodate your baby. Breastfeeding stimulates the production of oxytocin, which makes the uterus contract. If you're finding these pains tiresome, focus on the positives; they don't last long and you are on the way back to a flatter stomach!

The importance of skin to skin

That first cuddle with your wet, warm, wriggly baby is the moment you dream of during your pregnancy, but there's actually more to it than just an embrace. There is a surprising amount of research to show that direct skin-to-skin contact in the hours following birth has fantastic benefits for both mother and baby. Having nested quite happily in your uterus, it's quite stressful being squeezed out of the birth canal and being born, and skin-to-skin contact has been shown to be comforting to new babies. Numerous studies have shown that babies who had early skin to skin after birth were calmer, less stressed and cried less in the ensuing 24 hours than babies who had none; their heartbeats were slower and, hours later, they were warmer and more likely to breastfeed better.

If for some reason your baby can't have skin to skin with you, experiencing that contact with the father has similar benefits. In some rare cases the baby has to have important medical intervention that means skin to skin is impossible. If this is the case, focus on the amazing things that are being done to save your baby's life. Not having skin to skin doesn't mean you will not bond with or breastfeed your baby. Our message to you is that if it's possible, it's really worth doing.

Being able to feed your baby is obviously one of the most important things to learn and, as a result, the midwives are keen to help. They generally won't let you leave hospital until your baby is latching on well. Unfortunately a lot of advice given about breastfeeding is contradictory and this can be really frustrating for new mothers. If you're struggling to breastfeed you can be made to feel like you're falling at the first hurdle – and being told you are 'doing it wrong' when you are just following the advice of the previous midwife can be immensely frustrating and emotional. Try not to become despondent and, instead, focus on following advice from just one person.

Although midwives are brilliantly trained in delivering babies, and some have huge knowledge around breastfeeding, they might not all have been specifically trained in helping women (and babies) breastfeed. If you're not finding the advice you are getting is working, ask to see a breastfeeding specialist, which most hospitals provide. There are also some great books written by people who have dedicated their careers to helping women breastfeed, as well as a number of apps and videos; these can hugely help women who are struggling. It's worth going to an antenatal breastfeeding class before you've had your baby so that you understand the basics.

If you've had a caesarean

For those who have had a caesarean, it's not always possible to have skin-to-skin contact and a feed right away. Because you're on an operating table being stitched up, lying flat with a screen at your chest, a lot of women find it hard to hold their baby securely while in this position. It's worth asking your midwife if you can leave one arm out of the hospital gown so that your baby can have skin-to-skin contact on your chest – even if you can't actually start feeding your baby.

If you can't manage holding your baby, don't feel guilty about passing your baby to your partner. They should be able to sit right beside you. Encourage them to strip off their top and cuddle your baby close; whether it's your warmth and heartbeat your baby is hearing or your partner's, your baby will benefit and there will be plenty of time for cuddles and a first feed with Mummy afterwards.

The rest of the operation takes around 40 minutes and afterwards you're transferred to the recovery room for a few hours, where you'll be sitting more upright and be able to get going with that first feed.

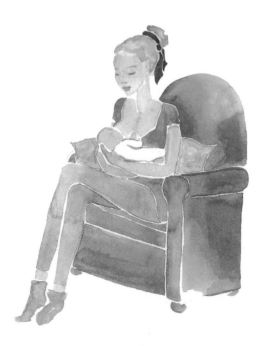

53 Your recovery *after birth*

Labour is called labour for a reason. Many women compare the lead-up (the pregnancy) to preparing for a marathon and the labour like the marathon itself. No matter how the marathon went for you, everyone needs to recover afterwards.

Even if your birth was extremely 'easy', it is common to feel exhausted, stiff and generally sore after giving birth. If you had a vaginal delivery your perineum will probably be swollen and uncomfortable, and if there have been stitches it may be a bit painful for the first few days.

> Don't be a hero; take enough painkillers to leave you pain-free. There are no prizes for bravery; indeed evidence has shown that you recover more quickly if you are not in pain. You will only be given painkillers that are safe for breastfeeding mothers.

 ## Your hospital stay
Generally wards are not conducive to getting much rest:
- The midwives are busy with people coming and going all night long and looking after the women on the ward. They need to do their job, and them doing so may mean you don't get much sleep.
- Your baby will be waking to feed at least every three hours. Even if your baby is not crying, the chances are that someone else's is, and the likelihood of you getting a good period of sleep is pretty slim.
- On top of that, some postnatal wards now allow fathers to stay the night, which is great for the mother but means double the amount of people in the ward. It can help to bring an eye mask and earplugs along with you. This will block out the majority of background noise but you will still hear your baby crying.

Easing post-birth discomforts

A sore perineum

- An ice pack, bag of frozen peas or cooling perineal pad can provide relief to this area.
- Try to avoid sitting directly on the perineum. Either lie on your side or use two rolled-up towels to sit on, taking the pressure off your perineum.
- It can really burn when you pee and the urine passes over the stitches. You can make this a lot more comfortable by using a jug to pour warm water over the area while you urinate.
- As long as you no longer have a catheter in, it is never too early to start doing your pelvic floor exercises after birth. Don't worry if you can't feel them initially, continue to do them and soon the

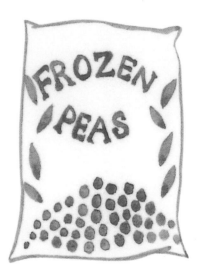

sensation will return. Doing your pelvic floor exercises will increase blood flow to the perineum, aiding recovery. If you still can't feel them a few weeks after birth, then have it checked out by a woman's health physiotherapist.

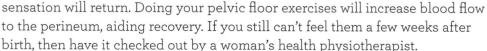

Haemorrhoids (or piles)

Even though these are fairly common in pregnancy and after a vaginal delivery, no one talks about these. Painful or itchy lumps coming out of your bottom, they are easily treated. They may develop in pregnancy or only after you have delivered, but the good news is they'll probably disappear on their own in the first few weeks after you've delivered. You can use over-the-counter treatments and ice packs to resolve them. Avoid becoming constipated as this just makes them worse, and try not to do any heavy lifting or straining. If they don't go away, see your GP, who can give you stronger medication or might recommend surgery.

Constipation

That first poo is quite often terrifying and referred to by some as 'the fourth stage of labour', so being constipated is something you can really do without. Unfortunately most women tend to get a little constipated because they're dehydrated from labour, haven't eaten much over the last 24 hours and the nervousness of pushing a poo out of this tender area, makes them 'hold it in'. Added to this, some pain-relief medications can make women constipated. So …

- Drink plenty of water throughout labour and rehydrate after delivery.
- Snack on high-fibre food and drink that will get your bowels moving.
- Even though you might feel anxious about opening your bowels, it's much better that you do a poo. Use a clean sanitary towel to support your stitches if you're worried about them.
- Take a stool softner, particularly if you've had any constipating medication.

 ## After a caesarean

Having a caesarean section is major abdominal surgery and there is no doubt that the recovery afterwards is much harder than after a vaginal delivery.

You will be encouraged to get up and out of bed in the first 12–24 hours after the operation, and this has been shown to aid recovery. Getting out of bed and walking for the first time will be very uncomfortable. You will be hunched over and will need someone walking next to you supporting you. You will also need help having a shower and putting clothes on – your midwife will help you with this. Your tummy will hurt when you do almost anything – move, laugh, sneeze, poo or sit up. It will be difficult to pick your baby up out of the cot without help and, although the midwives will do their best to assist you, it is a good idea to have someone with you as much as possible to help with little things.

The good news is that it gets better very quickly. By day two most women feel significantly better and by day three there is a similar improvement again. By the time you go home you will still be walking a bit gingerly and the ride home in the car will be a bit uncomfortable, particularly over any bumps, but you will be feeling much more like yourself.

You will be offered painkillers both in the hospital and to take home with you. If you are in pain, take them! You are more likely to need them once you get home as you will be more active so make sure you are discharged with enough. Beware though that some of the painkillers, particularly those containing codeine, are constipating.

If you had a similar operation for anything other than childbirth you would probably be off work for a couple of weeks. With a caesarean you have a baby to look after and will want to do a lot more than you should. It is really important to take things easy and not to push your body. It might be worth thinking about extra help, be it from family and friends or a professional if that is an option (see page 100).

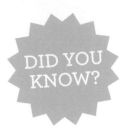

It is common to get stomach cramps after a caesarean. This is usually trapped wind and will not last long. Shoulder pain is also a common symptom and it is caused by diaphragm irritation during the operation.

A few post-caesarean rules

- Having had a caesarean does not mean you can forget about your pelvic floor exercises. Start doing these as soon as your catheter is out.
- Do not drive for six weeks (you will feel like you can but for insurance reasons you can't).
- You should not lift anything heavier than your baby for six weeks. This includes your baby in the car seat or up and down stairs in the pram. You will feel like you can but if you push it in the early days it can slow down your recovery and make long-term complications more likely.
- You can start gentle exercise if your doctor is happy with your recovery after your six-week check (see below). This does not mean running around the park the day after your six-week check. Take it slowly to avoid any damage.

Hospital checks for you and your baby

The midwives and doctors will want to do some daily checks on you and your baby in hospital and these will include:

You	Your baby
Feeling your tummy to check the uterus is contracting properly	Checking for jaundice
Checking your bleeding to make sure it is not too heavy or unusual	Weight check
Checking your scar if you have had a caesarean	Umbilical cord stump check – to ensure it is not getting infected
Checking any perineal swelling or stitches	Hearing test
Blood tests to check your haemoglobin before you leave	

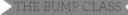

Your baby should be checked by a paediatrician or specially trained midwife before you leave the hospital and they may give you iron tablets to go home with.

 ## Bleeding

Regardless of whether you've had a caesarean or vaginal delivery, you will bleed for around four to six weeks after the birth of your baby. This painless bleeding is the lining of the uterus shedding itself – not damage caused during labour! For the first few days it will be very heavy, generally much more so than a period, and you will need to wear heavy-duty maternity pads. After a couple of weeks it will slow down and you may be able to use regular sanitary pads. You should not use tampons in this time. Let your midwife or doctor know if there are any sudden changes in the bleeding, such as sudden clots or change in volume or smell.

 ## Returning home

Most women are relieved to be leaving hospital and excited to be taking their baby home for the first time. It is common to feel anxious. Every new parent does. The enormity of the situation hits you that you have a new baby with no instruction manual! Don't worry – you will learn very quickly.

Only a generation ago (and it is still the case in many European countries), it was standard practice to stay in hospital for a week or so after a normal delivery, recovering physically, learning how to look after your baby and establishing feeding. Nowadays some women are discharged as early as six hours after birth, going back home, where it is much harder to recover and be looked after.

For this reason we advise getting back into your nightwear as soon as you get home. Although you don't need to be confined to your bed, being in your pyjamas will encourage your 'recovery mode' and make you less likely to overdo it. Stay in your pyjamas and don't leave the house for, at the very least, three or four days after leaving hospital.

54 Your *newborn baby*

Your baby will have two soft spots on the top and back of her head. These fontanelles are where the baby's skull bones have not yet met. The one at the back closes quite quickly. The one at the top might not close for 18 months or so.

Caucasian babies usually have blue eyes when they are born. If this is going to change, it usually does so in the first six months, but it can change up to a year after birth. Asian or Afro-Caribbean babies usually have brown eyes when they are born.

Your baby may have some bruises or marks from the birth. These will settle quickly.

The cord remnants still attached to the baby will shrivel up and usually fall off within the first 10 days of life. (For cord care, see page 175.)

Your baby may have a slightly elongated head from being squeezed through the birth canal. This settles in a few days.

Immediately after birth babies are wet and covered with the vernix that has been protecting their skin in the womb. They may be a little bloody. They will be rubbed down by the midwife after birth, but not usually bathed until a few days later.

You may notice that your baby may look a little cross-eyed. This is perfectly normal, as babies are not able to focus very well in the early days; this usually settles within a few weeks.

Swollen genitals (see page 165).

Many babies are born with birthmarks, which are skin blemishes, often caused by clusters of small blood vessels under the skin.

Types of birthmarks
- **Stork marks:** These marks on the forehead and back of the neck are common on Caucasian babies. (The implication from the name is that they are the mark left by the stork carrying your baby while delivering her to you – if only it were so easy!) These usually disappear within a year.
- **Strawberry naevus:** These are moles of various sizes that look a bit like a strawberry. Some increase in size for the first year and then shrink. They usually disappear by five years.
- **Mongolian blue spots:** These are a flat, darker patch of skin, sometimes looking a bit like a bruise. They are common in dark-skinned babies on their backs or buttocks. They usually fade in the first two years.
- **Port wine stains:** These are dark red marks flat to the skin, which rarely fade.

 ## Blame the hormones ...

Little baby girls and boys may be born with swollen breasts, and in some cases they may even leak milk. This usually only lasts a few days and, once again, you can blame your hormones. These can also cause a little bit of vaginal bleeding in baby girls.

Baby boys will normally have extremely large testicles after birth and often it is the first thing that parents notice (particularly the fathers, who are keen to tell the midwives that this baby is indeed 'my boy'). In fact the size of a newborn's testes is not genetic but, once again, it is hormone-related. Little girls have swollen genitals for the same reason. Both settle within a few weeks.

 ## Newborn checks

Immediately after birth your baby will have a preliminary examination by the midwife. However, before you are both discharged home, your baby will have a newborn check. This is a full, top-to-toe examination by a paediatrician or specially trained midwife. Any concerns will be raised with you, but it's a good opportunity to ask any questions you might have.

Your baby will be given a quick and painless test to check her hearing. This is usually done when you are still in hospital, but if not will be done in the first few weeks. You will be given the results immediately.

Special-care babies

Occasionally a newborn baby will be taken off to the special-care baby unit or the high-dependency unit if there are any concerns about her after she is born. This is obviously really hard for the parents, and they always imagine the worst.

Every situation is different but try to remember that the medical staff usually have a very low threshold for admitting babies they have concerns about. A lot of babies will only spend a short period of time being closely monitored and having some tests done before they join their mother again. If you are in this situation, try to be positive and think how lucky your baby is to have this expert help at hand to look after her. You will be encouraged to express colostrum to give her. Usually the staff will allow parents to spend as much time with their baby as they like.

If your baby needs to stay in hospital once you have been discharged, you can either go home and visit during the day or many hospitals have a patient hotel you can stay in.

'When Ludo was born he had to spend a few days in special care because he had a punctured lung. Seeing him in his little cot with a feeding tube in his nose and a drip in his hand was awful. When I walked in and found them doing a brain scan I thought something terrible had happened. I asked them about it, and they told me that they routinely do brain scans on all babies that are admitted and that there was nothing to worry about. I learnt that doctors are never not going to tell you their concerns; they will always be honest. Ludo left special care after a couple of days and thrived. Today, as I watch my exuberant five year old climbing trees or chasing his sister in the park, I find it hard to remember those worrying days, but I'm so grateful that he had the best care possible where the medics were concerned.' MARINA

Jaundice

While on the postnatal ward you may notice a few babies lying under a sun lamp with only their nappy on and little eye masks protecting their eyes. These babies are being treated for jaundice, a condition that makes the skin and the whites of the eyes go yellow. It typically starts at days two to three and lasts until around day ten. If it starts earlier or goes on longer your baby may need additional treatment. If your baby has jaundice, once you are at home it is a good idea to put her basket under a window, where the sunlight will help to break down the pigment bilirubin that causes the jaundice.

55 The first night at home
with your baby

Your baby will arrive home in a car seat, but once at home she needs to sleep flat on her back. She will need to be with you for at least the first few weeks rather than in a room on her own, so most parents use a Moses basket, which is small and portable. Babies usually like the secure feeling of being in a little basket. However, it is also fine for your baby to be in her cot right from the beginning if she is happy there.

The first night alone with your baby is a whirlwind of emotions. You're proud, relieved and overwhelmingly happy, but also thoroughly exhausted.

Encourage your partner, just for this night, to be with you during the night feeds. After the first night, there is probably no need for you both to be awake during night feeds, but on the first night, when you might be feeling out of your depth and nervous of your abilities as a mother, it is really useful.

'Despite supposedly having some knowledge ... I didn't sleep a wink the first night at home with our daughter.' YIANNIS (CONSULTANT PAEDIATRICIAN)

Your noisy newborn
Newborn babies are often very noisy. Their airways have been filled with fluid while in the womb and, although most of this will have cleared with the first few breaths, there tends to be a lot of coughing, vomiting, snuffling, sputtering and sneezing in the early days, as she tries to clear the remaining fluid. This will probably cause you to have some minor 'heart attack' moments when you are alone with your baby, particularly at night. Although the sounds they make are sometimes worrying for mothers, babies are in fact very adept at clearing their airways and don't usually need any help in doing so.

What to do if your baby won't settle:

It's not uncommon for babies who have slept soundly for the first day or two to suddenly wake and simply refuse to settle, and the constant crying can prompt their anxious and exhausted parents to question whether they are fit for parenthood.

Here are some steps to follow that might help soothe your baby:
- Check she is not hungry, wet, dirty, too hot or too cold.
- Try to wind her (see page 194).
- Swaddle her (see page 226).
- Jiggle her around or rock the crib. (Having been carried by her mother for nine months, she is used to movement and the sound of a beating heart, so these will often soothe her.)
- Some babies find sucking very soothing – try a dummy or your little finger.
- Some babies are born particularly hungry. If your baby simply won't stop screaming, you have tried breastfeeding and nothing else is working, it is possible that she is hungry and is not getting enough breast milk to satisfy her. In this situation, you can try giving her some formula milk. This will often do the trick and it doesn't mean that you won't be able to breastfeed. On the contrary, if you're relaxed and content that your baby is happy, you'll be much more likely to establish successful breastfeeding.

Bear in mind that persistent crying can sometimes (albeit rarely) suggest illness, so if your baby really won't settle, get her checked by your doctor.

'It is not uncommon in paediatric Accident and Emergency for a mother to bring her newborn – who won't stop crying – back to hospital, concerned that there is something dreadfully wrong. More often than not, the baby will settle with a bottle of formula, which is kept in the A&E department for this very purpose. Mothers are encouraged to continue breastfeeding regularly, bearing in mind that the baby might still need 'top ups' with formula for a day or two until the mother's milk supply is more established. Needless to say, if the feeding doesn't settle your baby and you have concerns, you should seek medical advice.' CHIARA

Dos and don'ts

- Do have a good home-cooked dinner; you need to keep your energy levels up if you're breastfeeding and home-cooked food on your own crockery will be heaven after hospital food. But don't spend hours in the kitchen yourself!
- Don't be tempted to invite everyone over to toast your baby's birth. Wait until you've rested and can actually enjoy it.
- Do go to bed early; this could be a long night.
- Don't decide it's time to reorganise the nursery.
- Do avoid cracking open the champagne; breastfeeding mothers often find champagne gives their babies wind, making them uncomfortable.
- Do drink lots of water; put a big bottle by your bed and make sure you've got one to hand while you're feeding, along with some snacks.
- Do have your baby sleeping next to you.
- Don't worry about every snuffle and grunt your baby makes, although it will be hard not to.

DID YOU KNOW?

Many mothers worry about their babies choking on their vomit if they put them to sleep on their backs. There is no need to worry. Babies turn their heads to the side when they vomit, even during their sleep.

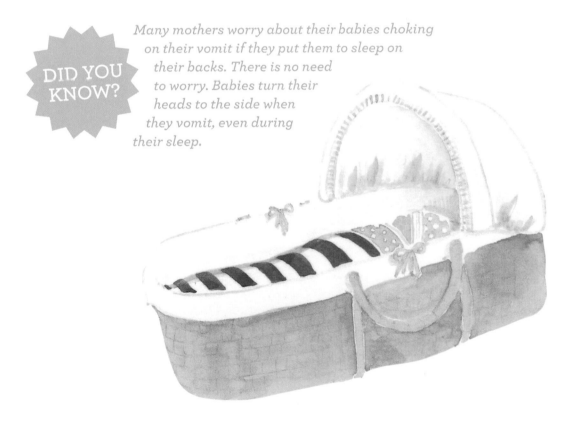

56 Your baby's *first year*

1st MONTH

At around two weeks she'll start to wake up, becoming more fun but also more demanding …

During the first few days your baby might lull you into a false sense of security, sleep lots and feed the WHOLE time.

Watch out! Around days three to five your milk comes in and the baby blues hit. Be prepared for a flood of unexplained emotions.

2nd MONTH

At around six weeks your baby will finally give you a well-earned smile … and you'll realise that every sleepless night has been worth it.

At six weeks your baby will have a check with the GP and you will also have your postnatal check.

By now you can start to think about exercising again … gently.

Your baby should be able to hold her head up and face forward in a baby carrier – which they generally LOVE!

By month three many mothers have started introducing a gentle routine. This can make your life easier and encourage your baby to sleep longer at night.

3rd MONTH

You might start thinking about sex in this month again … but don't forget CONTRACEPTION.

At eight weeks she has her first set of immunisations.

At 12 weeks she will have her second set of immunisations.

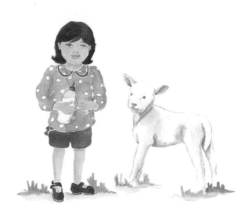

4th MONTH

She will start to squeal with laughter.

At 16 weeks she will have her third set of immunisations.

5th MONTH

She will start to push herself up on her arms and start to love toys, mirrors, etc.

6th MONTH

Once your baby is six months old she should start eating solids. Most babies love the new tastes and textures, and this is a great time for your baby to explore.

At around six months your baby will probably be able to sit up. Enjoy this magical time when they can play but not move ...

Most babies will get their first tooth around this month – although some get teeth as early as two months and some as late as ten.

7th MONTH

By seven months you can start introducing protein into your baby's diet. Most babies are delighted to progress from carrot to chicken.

....

If you haven't already, it's time to introduce finger foods – a baby rice cake is a great way to keep a fractious baby entertained.

....

8th MONTH

Once your baby is well established on solids she should no longer need feeding at night.

You'll probably be nearly back to your normal size by now, but a lot of women will still have a bit more weight to lose. Dig out those skinny jeans and make a last effort to fit back into them.

> Once she's on finger foods, the risk of choking becomes much more real. It's crucial that you know what to do if this happens – do a paediatric first-aid course.

Your baby might start to pull herself up; it's not long now until she walks. The danger zone has now increased ...

10th MONTH

Most babies are starting to crawl around this time. This opens up a world of excitement for your baby. Make sure your house is safe for her!

9th MONTH

Some babies start to develop separation anxiety. Be reassuring but know that this is entirely normal and soon passes.

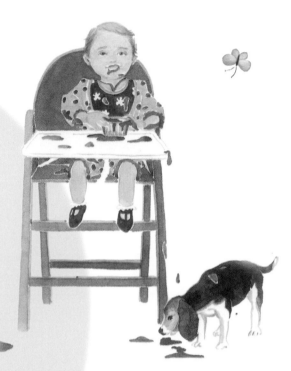

11th
MONTH

She will be able to understand a lot you say by now, even though she won't be able to talk.

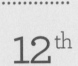

Babbling might turn into first words; it might be 'Mama', although it's usually 'Dada', as it's easier to say!

12th
MONTH

Hurray, you've made it through the first year! This celebration is more for the parents than the baby.

First steps can take place any time from 10 months to 18 months. Don't hurry but encourage. Be aware that once she learns to walk, nothing will be the same ...

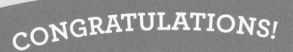

CONGRATULATIONS!

57 You and your baby in the *first two weeks*

The first couple of weeks after your baby is born is usually a magical time. Providing your baby is well, she will probably spend most of the time sleeping, waking every 3-4 hours for a feed. After a feed, she will probably spend a short amount of time awake before falling asleep again, and so the cycle continues.

Newborn babies don't need to be 'entertained'. Just being in the world is stimulation enough and your baby will be busy processing all the new sights, sounds and smells around her in the short spells she is awake. Sleep is key for her brain development and she really can't have enough of it. As long as she is waking for feeds, feeding well and is alert when she is awake, you don't need to worry that your baby is sleeping too much. Don't be scared of picking her up, cuddling her and getting to know her right from the beginning.

Parents are often lulled into a false sense of security in those early days and think 'What is all the fuss about – this is easy!' Just as those thoughts are going through their mind, babies often wake up and become a bit more challenging!

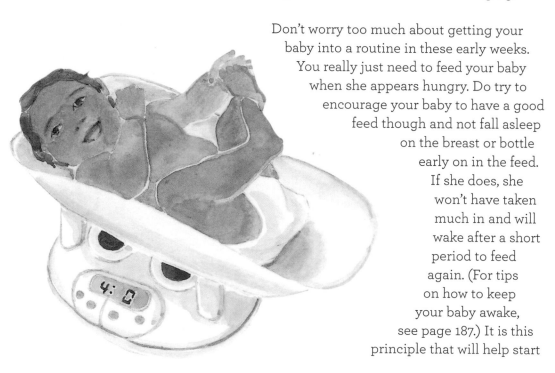

Don't worry too much about getting your baby into a routine in these early weeks. You really just need to feed your baby when she appears hungry. Do try to encourage your baby to have a good feed though and not fall asleep on the breast or bottle early on in the feed. If she does, she won't have taken much in and will wake after a short period to feed again. (For tips on how to keep your baby awake, see page 187.) It is this principle that will help start

Cord care

The umbilical cord stump will usually fall off when your baby is 7–10 days old. Until then you need to keep an eye on it and check it's not becoming infected. It can look a bit disgusting and start to smell towards the end. This is normal. Keep it clean with cooled boiled water and cotton wool. If the skin around it starts to look red, or it doesn't appear to be healing, see your doctor.

When your baby still has her umbilical cord stump, there is no hard and fast rule about whether the nappy should cover it or be strapped underneath. It depends on what you feel works best for your baby.

As it starts to come off, resist the temptation to pull it off. Just leave it be. It might be slightly raw looking for a few days but mostly it will heal nicely, leaving a perfect little tummy button.

the beginnings of a gentle routine. However, in the early weeks you do need to be guided by your baby and, as a rule, you should always offer her milk if you think she might be hungry.

 ## Your baby's weight

Weight is an issue that new mothers are often obsessed with. Not theirs (well, probably theirs too!) but the baby's. It is normal for breastfed babies to lose up to 10 per cent of their birth weight in the first week because your milk doesn't come in for a few days. Once your milk comes in, they should then start steadily putting on weight.

The midwives and health visitors will be keeping a close eye on your baby's weight in that first week, and if they have any concerns they will give you appropriate advice. If your milk comes in early and you have lots of it your baby may not lose any weight, but more often than not they do.

 ## What visits can I expect from my midwife/health visitor?

In the UK it is normal practice for a midwife to visit you at home the day after you are discharged from hospital. She will answer any questions and help you with problems you may be experiencing. She should come again in the first week. Some women will need more support and may receive more frequent visits.

You will also be seen by a health visitor – a specially trained nurse who is attached to your GP practice. They will usually visit you at home at around day 10 after your baby is born and bring with them the red book (your child's health record, in which all vaccinations and healthcare encounters are documented). Afterwards they are available for advice and queries about your baby as they grow up, at a weekly baby clinic, usually at your GP practice.

 ## Checks in the first few weeks

As well as the initial newborn checks (see page 165), your baby will have some tests in the first few weeks:

Heel-prick test (or blood-spot test)

When your baby is five days old your midwife will weigh your baby and do a blood test. This is done by pricking the baby's heel and squeezing a few drops of blood onto a card. This is then sent to a laboratory for analysis. It can take a few months for the results to come back. Parents are only contacted if there is an abnormal result.

The heel-prick test checks for:
- Sickle-cell disease – a hereditary blood disorder
- Cystic fibrosis – a serious genetic disorder that seriously affects the lungs and intestines and is life-limiting
- Phenylketonuria (PKU) – a rare but serious disorder that can be treated but can cause mental disability if untreated
- Congenital hypothyroidism – a rare condition that can cause growth problems and mental disability if not treated early
- MCADD (medium-chain acylCoA dehydrogenase deficiency) – a very rare condition that is inherited and potentially life-threatening. Diagnosing it early can prevent serious illness.

58 Riding the emotional *rollercoaster*

If you thought you felt overly emotional in your pregnancy, be prepared for the first few weeks of your baby's life. Your emotions could well be all over the place – one minute you might feeling utterly elated, unable to imagine being happier, and the very next, totally overwhelmed by the magnitude of responsibility you now have and the realisation that nothing will ever be the same again. Do remember this is normal and, as you find your feet, your emotions will level out and you'll start to feel a bit more like yourself.

In those first weeks with their baby, most mothers say they feel excited and tremendously happy. For the first time they are a little family unit and, however you look at this, it's amazing. Often mothers feel an overwhelming love for the father of their child and incredibly proud of their baby, who, in their eyes, is the most beautiful baby they've ever seen.

Some mothers though, who might have expected to 'feel the love' immediately, find the adjustment a little harder. It's not surprising considering you've just been through labour and won't have slept for some nights. It doesn't mean you won't establish a bond with your baby; it sometimes just takes a little time. So don't worry about it – it will probably creep up on you when you least expect it.

> *'I had a tough labour and when I finally held my baby, I was delighted he was safe, but I didn't feel the overwhelming love I'd expected. We took him home, I was exhausted, overwhelmed and sore. On the second night, he woke at 3am and wouldn't go back to sleep. Crippled with exhaustion, I laid him on my lap and looked at him and suddenly, like a freak wave, I was engulfed with a feeling of pure love for my little boy.'* NATALIE, THE BUMP CLASS

You are also likely to be feeling the following:

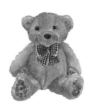

● Extremely tired: Don't underestimate the debilitating effects of tiredness (sleep deprivation is a very effective torture technique after all!) Girls regularly say this is the hardest part of motherhood. Forget the birth, any tearing or an episiotomy - dealing with lack of sleep is the real challenge (see page 230).

- Overwhelmed: Your life has just changed in the most monumental way and for many mothers and fathers the realisation of just how big this change is only hits them when their baby has arrived.
- Teary for no reason: The week after your baby is born, your body undergoes a massive hormonal change, and this often results in unexpected bouts of crying for no reason. It's probably at its most pronounced on about days three to five, when your milk comes in, and it even has its own name: 'the baby blues'. Even the most together, unemotional girls will suddenly be floored by how the most inconsequential thing will provoke uncontrolled sobbing. Don't resist the crying; it's part of your body's changing state, but reassure yourself that this is completely normal and that, in a week or so, you should be back to your normal self.
- Sore: Pain itself is exhausting, and, quite frankly, you'll be exhausted enough already without having to deal with unnecessary pain, so take enough painkillers.
- Sweaty at night: As if your nights weren't complicated enough at this stage, you will probably start sweating profusely at night. A huge number of girls have heard nothing about the night sweats before it affects them and they're perplexed at why they wake up drenched in sweat at night. Again this is to do with the hormonal changes in your body and usually happens at the same time as your milk comes in. It's relatively short-lived, and usually goes within about 10 days, but do be prepared for regular sheet and nightwear changes.
- Frustrated with your partner: Mixed with the adoration, frustration is very common. Because you're tired and hormonal, you're short-tempered, and sometimes partners can't do anything right! Try to warn them about this and ask them to be patient with you.
- Horrified about the way you look naked: The first time you look at yourself naked after the birth of your baby will be a real shock, and actually we advise that you don't submit yourself to this torture until you're more emotionally stable. Typically the day after you've had your baby, your tummy will still look about six months pregnant, but instead of that wonderfully taught baby bump that you so loved, it's floppy and flabby. Your skin will resemble crêpe paper and will be blighted by any stretch marks and possibly the linea negra. Your breasts will probably be enormous but not sexily voluptuous – more hard and almost square in their appearance. If you've had a caesarean, there will be a kind of shelf of skin over your scar; it probably means you won't be able to see the scar, which isn't a bad thing – it is red and angry at this stage. We don't want to terrify you

about what lies in wait, but it is torturous scrutinising yourself in the mirror at this stage, and there's simply no point in doing it. Leave it a week and the view will be a lot better; a week later, better still. So don't look but instead have a lovely shower and marvel at what a wonderful present your fabulous body has just given you.

'No one shared the delights of the night sweats with me before I had my baby and I was shocked by how much I could actually sweat at night. Sometimes I would wake three times a night, drenched in sweat to the extent that I would have to change my nightie, nursing bra and once even my sheets. I started sleeping with towels under me so that they could be changed more easily in the middle of the night.' MARINA

 ## Postnatal depression

This miserable condition affects more women than most think – 15–30 per cent of women suffer varying degrees, and it's something we feel all mothers should be aware of. It doesn't exclusively affect women who have previously suffered from depression, although this group are more prone to it. It does, however, have a tendency of creeping up on women who really didn't think they would be affected. For this reason, whatever your psychiatric background, don't disregard the likelihood of getting it.

The good news is that postnatal depression is usually easily treated; however, the key is to have it diagnosed early. The sooner treatment starts, the more quickly and efficiently it can be resolved. Watch out for the following signs:

- Persistent crying for no obvious reason (after the baby blues is over)
- Constant unhappiness and low self-esteem
- Difficulty bonding with your baby
- Neglecting yourself; not taking any pride at all in your appearance
- Not sleeping at night and being tired all day
- Seeming to lose a sense of time
- Losing your sense of humour; if you just can't see the funny side of things
- Extreme anxiety about your baby, despite reassurance
- Or, conversely, too little concern about your baby
- Sometimes, but not always, mothers might have negative thoughts towards their baby. This might not be as extreme as thinking of harming the baby but just being hyper-aware that you could.

YOUR EMOTIONS

Sometimes talking about your worries will make them better, and some women just need a few nights of good sleep, but sometimes it is a degree of postnatal depression, which once treated will make women feel like a different person.

If you are at all concerned, do not just ignore it and hope it will go away. The understanding, acceptance and therefore treatment of postnatal depression has come a long way in the last decade, and there are a range of treatments available to sufferers, such as talking treatments, hormone treatments and anti-depressants.

'I remember Chiara telling us about postnatal depression on The Bump Class and sitting there thinking that there was no way I was going to suffer. About four weeks after my baby was born I noticed I was especially teary and not really enjoying what I'd expected to be a magical time. My group were very honest about the challenges they were facing, but my situation just seemed more bleak than anyone else's and my days just seemed to have a black cloud over them. I looked back over my notes and recognised a lot of the symptoms. I went to see Chiara and just talking lifted a huge weight off my chest. We made a plan for treatment and once I walked out of her surgery I already felt my heart lift. The treatment was really effective and I've not looked back. I've since talked to many mothers who have suffered the same thing but didn't do anything about it. It's tragic that for some women the first years of motherhood were blighted by postnatal depression, and I'm so glad I was aware enough of the condition to recognise my symptoms.'
CLAIRE, THE BUMP CLASS

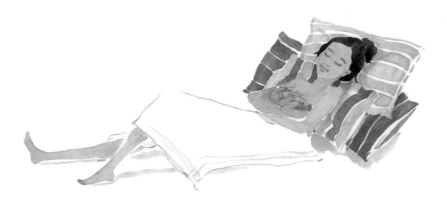

59 Basic *baby care*

 ## Safety

Healthy babies are pretty straightforward to look after as long as you follow certain rules.

The golden rules of baby safety
- Always put your baby to sleep on her back.
- Always support her head.
- Too cold is better than too hot.
- Never leave a baby alone on a high surface.
- Never take your eyes off a baby in the bath.
- Always use the pram brake or a wrist strap.

Babies cannot support their head on their own until about six to eight weeks, so supporting their heads is crucial. Babies don't regulate their temperature very well. If they are too cold they will cry; however, overheating is dangerous and has been linked with cot death. If in doubt, remember that too cold is better than too hot. Avoid hats indoors and, as a general rule, put your baby in one layer of clothing more than you are in (see page 220).

 ## Changing nappies

You will be amazed at how many nappies you go through in the early days. As a rule of thumb, you should change a nappy whenever it's wet or dirty, although they're so absorbent nowadays that, if you're out and about, a wet nappy can wait 30 minutes or so until you're in a convenient place to change it.

- When changing a nappy, make sure you've got everything you need to hand; you should never leave your baby unattended on the changing table, however immobile she may seem.
- For girls, wipe front to back – you don't want to get any poo in the vagina or urethra. For little boys, the direction doesn't matter.
- Most people use water and cotton wool in the early days but studies have shown

that there's no difference between using fragrance-free baby wipes and water. Although they're not great for the environment, wipes are far more practical than cotton wool and water, and you'll end up never leaving the house without them.

- When changing a nappy, make sure you have a muslin handy; the cold air often stimulates babies (mostly boys) to pee, and a muslin can stem the flow.
- When changing baby boys, make sure you point his penis down when you put the nappy on to prevent 'rising damp'.
- When your baby's bottom is clean, put a thin layer of barrier cream on it, and put a new nappy on. Don't worry about putting it on too tight – it's elastic so unlikely to be. Most new parents put them on too loose, which results in leakages ... they swiftly learn from their mistakes.
- Make sure you wash your hands thoroughly after every nappy change.

'My babies always seemed to get bored on the changing table so I stuck some black-and-white stickers to the shelf above it and my son was mesmerised. It meant he stayed still while I changed a nappy and loved his massage.' MARINA

 Nappy rash

This is caused by the irritant effect of urine and faeces and often affects little babies. A lot of babies have mild nappy rash, which is easily controlled:

- Change nappies frequently and as soon as you think they're wet.
- Make sure you clean your baby's bottom thoroughly; it's as important to give the whole area a clean after a pee as it is after a poo.
- Make sure your baby's bottom is as dry as possible. Pat it dry with clean muslin.
- Try to leave the nappy off as much as possible – put a towel down on the floor and let your baby have some nappy-free time when it's practical.
- Use a thin layer of barrier cream.

If the symptoms do not improve or worsen, see your GP. Some severe cases need to be treated with a medicated cream.

Cleaning your baby

Top and tailing

Most babies don't need a bath every day but they should be top and tailed. This is washing their face and neck (top) and their bottom (tail), using clean water and two separate vessels to hold the water for each task.

- Start with the head and, using separate pieces of cotton wool, clean each eye. Wipe the face, and clean the folds of the neck really well. As babies get bigger and fatter, milk and food dribble into these folds and it can get a bit cheesy and sore, so take time to clean it out really well.
- Clean under the arms. If your baby has lots of lovely rolls of fat, give them a good clean inside.
- Don't forget behind the ears; these can get scaly and sometimes infected.
- The bottom is really straightforward; just give it a good wash.

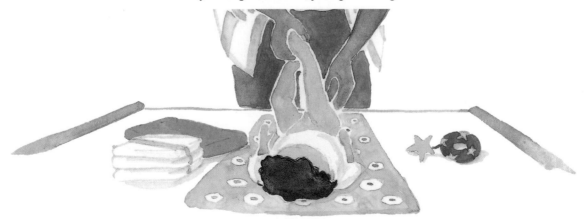

Bathing

Although baths aren't necessary every day, a lot of babies really love the bath and, as long as the water is not irritating her skin, there's no reason not to incorporate it into your evening routine. Remember that you should never take your eyes off your baby in the bath for a second. If you have to turn around to get anything, make sure you always have one hand on your baby.

- Get a simple plastic bath seat (we like the moulded plastic ones that you put in the bath as they hold the baby quite securely).
- A baby's bath should obviously not be too hot – a little warmer than lukewarm, but not as hot as your bath. That said, anxious mothers often run baths on the cold side for their babies, which the babies understandably don't like. A lukewarm bath quickly turns cold, so if you're finding your baby is whingey in the bath, try adding a little more warm water.
- Having a bath with your baby is lovely. Make sure there are two of you there – it makes it easier if you have someone to hand the baby to when you get out.
- After the bath, spend some time massaging your baby. You can use any kind of oil – olive oil works a treat. Babies tend to love being massaged, and it's a great way of cleaning in between those delightful folds of fat as they get older. It's a great time to interact with your baby. Ideally do it on your changing table so you're not straining your back and make sure the room is nice and warm.

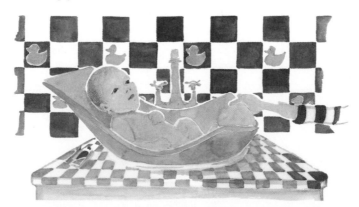

60 Breastfeeding

For some women breastfeeding comes easily; their baby latches on instantly and they never look back. For others it is a battle from day one. Try as they might, their baby struggles to feed from the breast and mothers often end up feeling that they've failed at one of the first fundamental tasks of motherhood.

Many people are passionate that all mothers should breastfeed and that's because it has undisputed benefits including:
- Protecting your baby against infections and diseases
- Helping you bond with your baby
- Protecting against cot death
- Reducing the likelihood of obesity
- Protecting against allergies including eczema
- Preventing constipation in babies
- Protecting the mother against breast and ovarian cancer
- Helping mothers lose weight (it uses about 500 calories a day)

Added to this, from a practical point of view:
- It's free
- It's hassle-free (no sterilising, no bottles)
- It's readily available at the right temperature with no chance of going off

For these reasons alone it's worth finding out about breastfeeding and seeking professional advice from a breastfeeding specialist if you find yourself struggling.

 ## Successful latching

As soon as possible after your baby is born, you will be encouraged to have some skin-to-skin time. Newborn babies have an incredibly strong urge to start feeding and she might well be able to manoeuvre herself to your nipple and start sucking in the first hour of life (see page 156). For many, the baby latches on and they never look back; it's as simple as that. For some, however, breastfeeding is mind-blowingly painful, and that is usually because the baby has not latched on quite right.

For a successful latch, ideally you want to aim your nipple for your baby's nose, encouraging her to open her mouth as wide as possible and take as much of the areola (the circular area around the nipple) into her mouth, with the actual nipple at the back of her mouth. The areola is tougher than the nipple; what you want is your nipple at the back of your baby's mouth, with her tongue on the areola.

It is important that she gets more of the areola close to her lower lip, so you are aiming for an off-centre latch. When she scoops up more areola close to her lower lip, your areola lies on her tongue and your nipple is right at the back of her mouth, out of harm's way. To help you understand this, pretend your thumbnail is your nipple for a moment and place your lower lip on the cuticle, then tip your thumb into your mouth and give it a suck. You will feel your tongue roll over the tip of your thumb and it really isn't very nice. This is what a shallow latch will feel like to a baby, and you can see how easily your nipple can become damaged. Now pop your lower lip on your thumb knuckle and tip your thumb into your mouth and give it a suck. You can feel that your thumbnail is right at the back of your mouth. This is what a deep latch will feel like to your baby and you can see how it will be more comfortable for you too.

Once your baby is latching on correctly, breastfeeding feels wonderful. At the beginning you'll feel quite cautious, wanting to make sure you're in the right position with all the right support but do try different positions and be adventurous as it will make breastfeeding easier.

Unfortunately some women, try as they might, find breastfeeding just doesn't work for them and their baby. We'd always suggest seeking professional advice before deciding to stop. Most hospitals will have a dedicated breastfeeding specialist who will offer great support and will often solve problems. There are also some great private breastfeeding specialists who will support you at home. If you've tried everything and nothing is working, then bottle-feeding is a great alternative (see page 190).

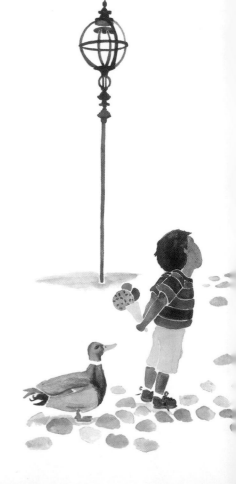

How to keep your baby awake while feeding

One of the hardest things about breastfeeding is that it's the perfect opportunity for your baby to have a little snack and then go back to sleep, as she's close to your warm body. Ideally you want your baby to take big feeds so that she learns to go longer in between each feed, sleeps longer and better and is generally happier when she's awake.

If you're finding she's falling asleep try:

- Taking a layer off her. She won't get too cold, as your body heat will keep her warm, but hopefully she'll be cool enough to stay awake.
- Tickling her feet or ear.
- Putting a little pressure on your breast, squirting more milk into her mouth, as this often wakes a baby up.
- Changing her nappy. A two-part feed with a bit of winding and a nappy change midway through is a good and practical way to get a baby ready for her second helping.

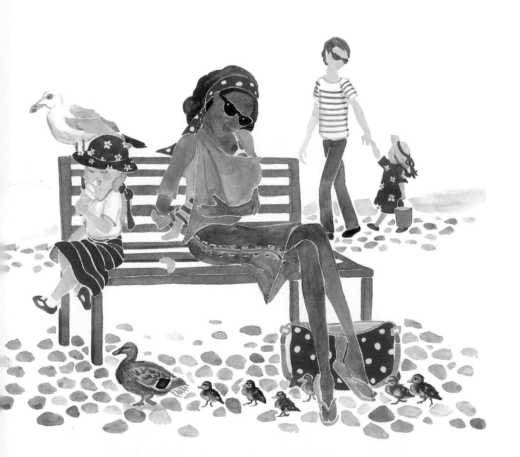

> **Q&A**
>
> *'How do my breasts know how much milk to produce?'*
> Breasts are clever things. Firstly they produce colostrum, the
> nectar that provides your baby with unique antibodies in the first
> few days of her life (see page 156). They then produce loads of milk
> on about day three when your baby is really hungry. This is essential as your
> breasts don't know whether you have one, two or three babies to feed and
> how hungry they will be. Your breasts respond to demand, so after a few
> days they will start adjusting the milk supply to what is being consumed.
> Obviously this varies hugely from woman to woman; some women
> overproduce milk and are at higher risk of mastitis and some struggle to
> produce enough and may have to top up with formula. Try not to overthink
> breastfeeding – after an initial teething period, for the majority of women
> it's straightforward and the easiest way to feed your baby.

 ## How often should you feed your baby?

As a general rule, newborn babies need to feed at least every three hours, although
some bigger babies might be able to stretch to four if their mother has lots of milk.
Sometimes newborn babies are very sleepy and might go longer between feeds; if
this is the case it's important to wake them for feeds as their drowsiness could be a
medical problem.

 ## How much should you feed your baby?

Unfortunately there is no gauge on the breast, nor on the baby, for us to know
accurately how much milk they've had. This is a bit of a design flaw. However, you
generally know your baby has had enough milk by the following:
- Feeling your breast to see if it has emptied; you'll work this out pretty quickly
  – a full breast feels hard and full and once emptied it feels soft and empty.
- After being burped, your baby is not interested in latching on and will
  happily settle.
- Looking at what comes out the other end (see The Spectrum of Poo, page 214)
- In the longer term, your baby's weight gain is a good indicator of how well
  she's feeding.

188

THE BUMP CLASS

We can't tell you exactly how frequently your baby should be fed or how long she needs to feed for. Babies and breasts vary hugely and therefore there is no one answer. Try not to worry too much; as long as your baby is settling well and growing as she should, you are doing brilliantly.

 ## How to stop breastfeeding

Whether you decide to stop breastfeeding at three months or three years it is a good idea to have a plan in place to gradually reduce it rather than going 'cold turkey'. Stopping breastfeeding too quickly increases the chances of you developing mastitis (see page 239). Once babies are established on three solid meals a day they need less milk so the baby will, to some extent, initiate the slowing-down process. Therefore weaning a three-month-old baby will take a longer time than weaning a one year old. There is a lot of advice out there on this topic but here are some general rules:

- Most importantly, take it slowly.
- Write down all the feeds that you do over a 24-hour period.
- Drop one feed every two to three days, or longer depending on how much milk you are producing.
- Space out the feeds that you drop. For example, if you are feeding at 7am, 11am, 3pm, 7pm and 11pm, you could start by dropping the 11pm, then the 11am, then the 7pm, then the 3 pm, and finally the 7am.
- Try to work out when your milk supply is at its highest and lowest. For many women the time when they have the highest milk supply is in the mornings (after a good night's sleep) and it's lowest in the evening (after a full day). The first feed to drop is when your milk supply is at its lowest, and the last feed to drop should be when it's at its highest.
- To slow down your milk supply at your chosen feed, you can either feed for a shorter time and then top your baby up with formula, or you could express the feed completely and reduce the amount of milk you express over a few days, until you no longer need to express at that time.
- If you find you are getting blocked ducts or sore breasts having dropped a feed, try expressing a little by hand in the bath or shower; this usually takes the edge off it.
- There are drugs available to stop your milk supply, but stopping naturally is easy if done correctly and is the technique generally recommended by health professionals.

61 Bottle-feeding

We've covered the benefits of breastfeeding in the last chapter; however, for some women, breastfeeding doesn't or can't work for whatever reason. If breastfeeding is not right for you, don't beat yourself up about it; formula is not harmful and your baby will still be getting what she needs. Focus on enjoying your baby and bonding with her during feeds, whether she's being fed from a bottle or from the breast.

Even if breastfeeding is working a treat, it's worth introducing a bottle of expressed breast milk around the time your baby reaches two weeks old. Babies quickly develop habits which they are very averse to changing. If you only ever breastfeed, the danger is that, by the time your baby is four months old, she will simply refuse to take anything but the breast. This is obviously fine while you're around, but should you need to be away for a day or not be able to breastfeed for whatever reason, you're in trouble. It also means you're the only person that can feed your baby, and, believe us, most mothers could do with a little help to give at least one of the feeds. We've spoken to lots of girls who have really struggled trying to introduce a bottle, and the longer you leave it, the tougher it gets.

 ## How to give your baby a bottle
Whether your baby is getting expressed breast milk or formula from the bottle, the technique is the same:
- Most small babies will take the bottle very willingly.
- When you're holding your baby, make sure she's not flat; it's easier for her to digest her milk if she's slightly upright, and it's easier for her to control the flow of milk this way.
- A lot of babies will dribble as they feed so have a cotton bib on her and a muslin handy.
- A baby will need to be winded after either a breast- or bottle-feed (see page 194).

 ## Warming milk
Breast milk is body temperature so many mothers will want to warm their milk to the temperature that the baby is used to, although this is not strictly necessary.
- It's best to warm milk in a cup of warm water or bottle warmer. Before you give it to your baby, shake it well to make sure it's an even temperature, and test it on your wrist to make sure it's not too hot.

- Never reheat milk.
- Always discard any milk left over at the end of a feed. If your baby is a slow feeder, don't worry. Breast milk or freshly mixed formula can be kept at room temperature for an hour.

'One of the best tips The Bump Class gave me was to see if my baby was happy to drink room-temperature milk. Even though she had got used to warm milk while breastfeeding, when I introduced a bottle, Lily was not at all fussy about the temperature and it made my busy life on the go infinitely easier not having to think about warming her bottle.' ROSIE, THE BUMP CLASS

 ## Expressing breast milk

Expressing is not glamorous. Speaking from experience, we know that hooking yourself up to a breast pump and seeing milk extracted from your breasts into bottles will make you feel like a cow. That said, being able to delegate some of your baby's feeds is invaluable, and even those who approached expressing with trepidation, admit that they quickly recover from bovine comparisons, grateful for how much easier expressing makes their lives.

- Invest in a good breast pump; you can either rent or buy these, but it's also worth seeing if you can borrow one from a friend.
- There are a variety of different machines out there – from single hand-operated ones to motorised double pumps. For most new mothers, time and efficiency are paramount; often those who have gone with the simpler models find them too time-consuming and change to the more efficient motorised versions.
- Breasts respond to demand so it's important when pumping not to overstimulate your breasts. If you're expressing a feed, try to express the same or just a little bit more than your baby would usually drink rather than as much as you can get out.
- Some people will express after a feed to increase supply; this can work if you aren't producing enough milk, but make sure you're also eating well and resting lots, as these affect milk supply.
- Breast milk can be stored either in the fridge (for up to five days) or the freezer (for three months). Make sure containers are labelled with the date. Because liquids expand when frozen, it's also worth noting the amount. Rather than freezing big amounts, freeze small amounts. Once defrosted, milk needs to be used or thrown away within 24 hours.

- After expressing you will need to wash all the machine parts exposed to your milk thoroughly and then sterilise them.

 ## Using formula

There are lots of different formulas on the market and all are heavily regulated so it's safe to assume that all are good to use. We'd recommend making your life as easy as possible and choosing a formula that is widely available rather than one you can only buy in specialist stores. If you are suddenly caught short, it's reassuring to know that you can always get a carton.

- Always use cool boiled water.
- Prepare milk on a clean surface and always follow the mixing instructions.
- At the beginning of the day, boil the kettle and put the right amount of boiled water into each bottle to cool down, ready for each feed.

'Rather than faffing around with bottle warmers once I introduced formula, I got into the habit of adding a little bit of boiling water to my cool boiled water. So if I was doing a 7 oz feed, I'd boil 5 oz of water in the morning, let it cool and, before adding the formula, would add another 2 oz of boiling water to make it the perfect temperature.' MARINA

The joy of using a bottle is that you can see exactly how much milk your baby is drinking. Don't be surprised if her consumption occasionally increases or decreases slightly. Babies have growth spurts and often will spend a few days drinking more. That said, some days they just don't have as much of an appetite (like us). Try not to count every ounce and obsess if your baby hasn't consumed what you'd anticipated – remember mothers of breastfed babies can't count the ounces! Instead, look at her consumption over a few days. If your baby is off her milk altogether, you will need to see your doctor more quickly.

Similarly, if your baby is wolfing down too much milk, try pacing the feed. Some babies don't realise that they can stop to catch their breath, so you need to help them pace their milk intake. To do this, allow her to latch and swallow a few times, then pop the bottle out of her mouth and put the teat on her top lip. When she is ready to continue feeding, she will tip her head back and start sucking again.

When you're happy that your baby is taking a bottle well and easily, we recommend that you ask your partner to do the last feed at night – usually around 10–11pm. If you're using expressed milk, you can express at 9pm and then GO TO BED. That way you can have 2–3 extra hours' sleep before your baby needs to feed in the night.

Sterilising feeding equipment

When using bottles, hygiene is incredibly important. Milky surfaces are great places for bacteria to grow, particularly nasty bacteria which can make little babies quite ill, so it's imperative to wash and sterilise all bottles thoroughly. There are various ways of sterilising baby equipment, including great travel solutions, so think carefully about what suits your space, budget and lifestyle best.

The World Health Organization recommends sterilising until your baby is one year old. Of course, by the time they're six months old they're sitting up, grabbing whatever they can and sticking it in their mouths. By the time they're crawling, they will put all sorts of 'unsterile' things in their mouths, so many mums feel that they can get away without sterilising after six months. If you do this, make sure you wash the milky bottles really thoroughly, using very hot water and soap.

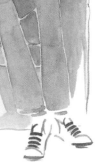

62 Winding

Regardless of whether you're breast- or bottle-feeding your baby, she will swallow a lot of air as she gulps down her milk. If this gets trapped in her tummy, it will cause considerable discomfort, so it's important that she's winded during and after a feed.

Winding will become a big part of your lives. For some babies, you simply sit them up and a nice, juicy burp will come up immediately and job done! For others, you'll sit them up, pat their backs, jiggle them around, put them on their tummies, pace up and down the stairs, sing 'the burp song' and, after an hour of this, finally a burp will come up. You might not always notice a burp but, if you then try to settle her or offer her a bit more milk and she's wriggly and unsettled, it's a good sign that there's still a burp in there. That said, if she settles nicely or starts to feed happily again, you can assume she's done all the burps she needs to ... for now.

Babies generally stop needing to be winded around the time they start sitting, at about six months old. It's not something that will suddenly stop; rather it will become easier and easier so you stop thinking about doing it and suddenly you realise that the burping procedure is something you no longer do.

TIP
Always make sure you have a muslin handy when burping, as a little bit of sick often comes up with the burp. And get into the habit of checking your clothes before you leave for work – a sure sign of a new parent is the telltale dribble of white spit-up on the shoulder!

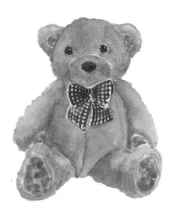

Winding positions

There are a lot of techniques for bringing burps up and you'll find that there are some that work for your baby all the time and some that don't work at all.

1. With your baby on your shoulder, her arms forward, patting her back.
2. Your baby sits on your lap, and you have the heel of one hand at the base of her back and the other hand supporting her head under her chin. You slowly rock backwards, upright and then forwards.
3. Your baby faces forward and your hand is over her body and tummy.

> *'Movement usually helps burping so you often see parents jiggling, bouncing, walking or even lunging! I found stairs brilliant for bringing up burps – but it had to be the actual stairs; as much as I tried to recreate the movement of going down stairs, it never worked as well.'* MARINA

Sometimes if you just can't get a burp up, try lying your baby down for a few minutes and then try burping her upright again. Often this will release that pesky air bubble.

1.

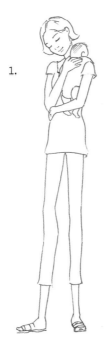

2.

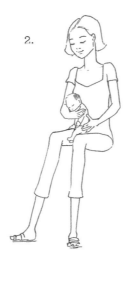

3.

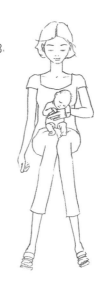

63 Why is my *baby crying?*

It is torture for a mother to listen to her baby crying. Until you're a mother yourself, you will not understand how each wail wrenches your stomach.

Not every cry means the baby is upset, uncomfortable or in pain. It is their only way of communicating and, as they get older, they'll cry when they're annoyed or frustrated as well. As you spend more time with your baby you will learn to identify her cries, and you'll soon realise that not all of them necessarily need responding to. Some babies grizzle a bit when they're going to sleep in their cot – some people believe that's just expelling a bit of energy before they go to sleep or even creating some background noise to help them get to sleep.

When your baby cries, the first thing to do is eliminate basic causes. More often than not one of these will be responsible and they are relatively simple to rectify.

The common causes

Hunger
With small babies you should always offer them food if you think they might be hungry. Some babies drink substantially more on some days than others, and that's because they have little growth spurts in the early days. When they're a bit older, it's a good idea to introduce a gentle routine to your baby's life. This will help you anticipate when she will be hungry.

Tiredness
If you watch them carefully, babies are good at giving us signs that they're tired. They might rub their eyes, yawn or turn their heads away. Little babies need a lot of sleep, and those that have enough sleep are generally more contented when they're awake. When your baby is a little older (around four to six weeks), introducing a gentle routine can give you a good idea of how much sleep your baby needs and when. Try to avoid multiple catnaps throughout the day; longer sleeps are more restorative and will result in a happier baby. The key is to avoid overtiredness. Very often overtired babies actually find it harder to go to sleep. This may be why babies who have not slept enough or well during the day will often sleep badly at night.

Being too cold

Feel the back of your baby's neck; if it doesn't feel nice and warm, try putting on an extra layer. Baby's hands and feet often feel cold, even when they're perfectly warm, so stick to her neck as a good indicator of temperature. Don't forget that overdressing your baby can be dangerous (see page 220).

Having a dirty/wet nappy

A dirty or wet nappy is pretty obvious. Babies are so different and some won't mind lying in a dirty nappy whereas others, particularly little girls, will scream in fury as soon as the nappy is a bit wet.

Wind

Even if she's had a good burp after her feed, there still may be another one in there. If you find she's wriggling uncomfortably when you put her down, try again to get the wind up. See page 194 for how to wind your baby.

 ## Evening fretting

You may well be reading this having tried all of the above. The chances are it's in the evening when you're in dire need of some peace, quiet and adult time. Annoyingly, this is often when babies are unsettled for no apparent reason. This even has its own name, 'evening fretting', and it is very common among small babies.

 ## What can you do?

- **Try feeding:** Even if you think she's had a good feed, it's common for mothers' milk supply to dwindle towards the end of an exhausting day. For this reason, the last feed of the day is commonly the first where mothers top up with some formula.
- **Try swaddling:** See page 226.
- **Try movement:** Don't worry about getting your baby into bad habits in the first few weeks – try rocking the crib, jiggling your baby, pushing her around the block in the buggy or even going for a drive. These early days are all about survival – you've got plenty of time to establish good habits.

If you're finding that her evening fretting is becoming habitual, try making the last hour of your baby's day all about winding down. Give her a bath and a nice massage, followed by her feed in a quiet, dark room. Then give her the last part of her feed while she's swaddled, ready for bed, and try to avoid eye contact with her. Bear in mind that eye contact for a new baby is very stimulating and, while it's lovely for you, it won't help her sleep.

Thankfully evening fretting is something most babies grow out of quite quickly so keep your spirits up; the chances are it will be a distant memory soon.

If your baby is crying for long periods and seems very uncomfortable, she might be suffering from colic or reflux. See page 201 for advice.

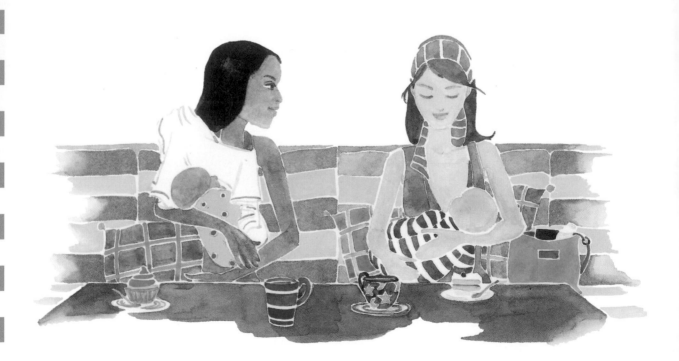

64 Understanding and communicating *with your baby*

Not being able to communicate effectively with your baby is definitely one of the things that makes parenthood more challenging. Crying might not necessarily mean she's in pain; it might be that she's frustrated, angry or simply just testing her vocal cords. Most new mothers don't feel that they can tell the difference between the types of cry. However, the more you actually listen to your baby's cries, the easier it will be to distinguish them. Rather than jump up and immediately react to a cry, try to take a minute to listen to it and observe any cues which might indicate what the problem is. This should allow you to work out what the various cries are, making being a mother so much easier.

 ## How to identify different cries

	Sound	Cues
Tiredness	A soft, moaning cry which almost has a rhythm to it. A lot of babies will use this cry to help them get to sleep, so resist the urge to rush to comfort your baby if you recognise this cry. Very often they're using this cry to expel energy or even to create their own white noise to help them get to sleep; rushing over to comfort them will only stimulate them and prevent sleep.	Rubbing of eyes and often ears, and later yawning. Turning her head to the side.
Hunger	A low-pitched cry that rises and falls. It often gets progressively louder. The only way to stop it is to feed your baby.	It's often combined with rooting (when the baby turns her head and opens her mouth in search of a nipple or teat) and her sucking her hands.
Discomfort	This is very different from a pain cry in that it's more whiney. Generally picking your baby up won't stop it – the only thing that will, is alleviating the discomfort, which might be a dirty nappy or colic.	Back arching or knees to chest and wriggling.
Pain	Often a sharp loud scream followed by silence (almost like the baby is catching her breath or even hyperventilating after the shock), followed by another loud, sharp scream.	Back arching can be a sign that they're uncomfortable and even in quite severe pain. It's often seen in babies with reflux (see page 202).

⭐ Talking to your baby

As crazy as it might sound, it's really important to start talking to your baby as if they're a little person from the moment you meet them. Not only will they find your voice reassuring and entertaining, but babies are like little sponges and the more they are talked to and communicated with from day one, the more likely they are going to be able to communicate with you in time. You may be surprised at how early your baby will start to communicate with you using little squeaks and sounds, often as early as a couple of months old. Before you know it they will be listening and beginning to understand..

I felt a bit silly talking to my newborn baby when clearly he had no understanding of what I was saying but I quickly got over it and it became a habit for me to just chatter away to him all day. I'd talk about anything, from changing his nappy to what I'd forgotten to buy. I found myself using a sing-song voice, which apparently mothers often do and is said to aid language development. Crucially though, I learnt not to be embarrassed about my chatter; I've no doubt that my baby benefitted both in the short and long term.' JESS, THE BUMP CLASS

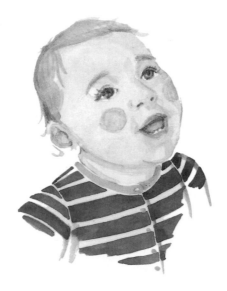

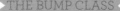

65 Does my baby have *colic or reflux?*

If your baby cries a lot more than seems normal and you feel she is uncomfortable with it, she may have colic or reflux. There is no accepted medical explanation for colic but it is generally thought to be due to a sore tummy, whereas reflux is medically explained. Colic tends to affect babies more in the evenings, and reflux affects babies all the time.

 ## Colic

How do I know if my baby has colic?
Babies with colic tend to scream explosively for prolonged periods with their knees drawn to their chest, and there is often no soothing them. By prolonged we mean continuously for 2–3 hours (although we appreciate that, for most addled mothers, a mere 5 minutes of screaming seems prolonged). Colic quite frequently affects babies in the evenings and it differs from evening fretting (see page 197) in that the babies are clearly quite uncomfortable rather than just whingey. Colic usually occurs from three weeks, peaks between six to eight weeks and thankfully tends to resolve by around 14 weeks.

 ## What can I do to help?
While there is no good evidence that colic is linked to diet, anecdotally breastfeeding mothers frequently associated it with various food types. Common culprits include:

- Garlic
- Spicy food
- Beans (and other foods that may cause wind in adults)
- Citrus fruits
- Coffee or caffeine products
- Dairy products

If you notice a correlation between colic and anything you're eating, it's worth eliminating things, one at a time, to see if it helps.

Over-the-counter medications are variably effective. It's worth talking to your pharmacist about what they might recommend and trying them one at a time.

Baby massage classes are not only a nice way for new mothers to socialise with their babies, but many babies with colic find this hugely soothing. A good instructor should give you tips on how to ease tummy pain at home.

A lot of Bump Class mothers swear by cranial osteopathy. Although evidence is scant, it does no harm and we see a lot of babies who appear to have been helped by it. If you do try this, make sure you see someone who is accredited and experienced in treating babies.

Babies with colic tend to prefer being on their tummies. This does not mean you should ever put them to sleep on their tummies. As tempting as this might be, it has a strong link to cot death (see page 228). Do however let your baby have lots of tummy time, which, as long as someone is watching her, is fine. They also like pressure on their tummy, so rocking them to sleep with their tummy on your tummy, or even putting something warm on their tummy, can really help; try a warm 'hot' water bottle or wrapping a muslin around their tummy for pressure.

Most babies grow out of colic by around 14 weeks so hang in there, but if you are worried about it in any way, see your GP.

> *My advice to parents of babies with colic is that if nothing seems to be working, it's really important for the mother to get time out from a crying baby. Give her to your partner, parent, willing friend or put her down safely in the cot while you take a deep breath. Remember, crying won't harm your baby.*
> *YIANNIS IOANNOU, CONSULTANT PAEDIATRICIAN*

 ## Reflux or silent reflux
What is reflux?
In some babies the valve at the top of the stomach that keeps the milk in once it has gone down is not quite strong enough so milk and stomach acid travel back up the oesophagus (swallowing tube), causing pain and discomfort. Remember all babies bring up some milk; if your baby is happy, content and gaining weight, this is not a concern.

What's the difference between reflux and silent reflux?
Reflux: In some babies the milk travels all the way up and causes them to vomit a lot of the time. Although this is messy and frustrating, babies who vomit with

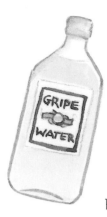

reflux tend not to be as uncomfortable, as the acidy milk has come out. However, it can mean that they don't put on weight, which is a serious problem so it does need treating.

Silent reflux: This is the term given to babies with reflux who don't vomit. As a result the acidy milk keeps on going up and down the oesophagus, which is painful and can be more challenging to diagnose. These babies are very uncomfortable and scream all the time but don't vomit more than normal babies.

What can I do to help?

The treatments for reflux and silent reflux are the same. Your doctor will advise on medications but there are also some practical things you can do:

- Keep your baby upright, particularly during and after feeds. You may find that putting her down in the car seat or bouncy chair for daytime naps helps. Similarly try raising the head of the cot or Moses basket by putting books under two of the legs.
- Feed little and often, particularly if your baby is vomiting a lot.
- If formula feeding talk to your doctor about using formula designed for reflux babies, which is thicker than normal formula. (Don't forget to change your bottle teats if you do this.)
- Reflux is sometimes linked to cow's milk protein allergy, especially if your baby also has eczema. In this case your doctor might recommend a cow's milk-free formula or, if breastfeeding, excluding cow's milk from your diet.
- A dummy can be very helpful for refluxy babies as it encourages them to swallow the acid back down.
- If breastfeeding, keep an eye on what you are eating and monitor if it appears to be affecting your baby.
- Cranial osteopathy is thought to be helpful in calming babies with reflux, as are some homeopathic medicines.
- Early weaning might be helpful; most paediatricians recommend weaning refluxy babies between four and six months, as this has been shown to improve their symptoms.

Talk to your doctor about medications for reflux. These are often very effective and will make your baby a lot more comfortable. Most babies will be on medication until they are well established on solids and sitting upright for most of the time.

'My second baby had reflux and, to be frank, the early months were an absolute nightmare. My first baby had been very easy, rarely cried and slept and fed well. My daughter was a completely different experience. There was no question of doing anything social as she cried constantly. Certainly in the first month there was rarely a time when she was awake and happy. She was either asleep, feeding or screaming and it was utterly exhausting. I felt awful for her as she was clearly in a lot of pain. She was started on medication at about six weeks and it made a huge difference. Even as a doctor, I, like every mother, did not want my baby to be on medication, but once she was on it, it was obvious that it had been the right decision. She was so much more comfortable and happy. That said, she still wasn't pain-free and continued to cry with some feeds. I would say that the next real turning point came at around six months when she was on three solid meals a day, after which she never looked back. She stopped her medication and the reflux has never been an issue since. As a result she is very tough and rarely cries with pain now that she is a toddler!' CHIARA

 ## Coping when your baby has colic or reflux

Having a baby with colic or reflux can make the whole experience of early motherhood much less enjoyable. It can make parents feel like they are doing something wrong and can be very demoralising – in some cases leading to depression. If you're experiencing this, try to share the load a bit to give yourself a break and do also talk about it frankly to your friends and family. If things are really bad, see your GP sooner rather than later; they will offer help for your baby and support for you.

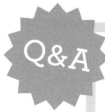

'Why does reflux seem to be more common now than in the past?'

Many paediatricians feel that this may be because we now put babies to sleep on their backs. Although we know this significantly decreases the risk of cot death, it may also be the reason we are seeing more reflux. Doctors are also better at diagnosing and treating the condition than they were in the past.

66 You and your baby *in weeks three and four*

On the one hand, by the time your baby reaches three weeks old, it will feel like you've been a mother for a lifetime, but on the other hand those weeks will have passed in a blur.

She may start to respond to noise and light; while most newborns are happy sleeping soundly anywhere, often the noisier the better, as they become more aware, their sleep may start to be disturbed. If you find this is happening, try putting her somewhere less noisy, especially once she's down in the evening. Often just outside the kitchen, where it might be quieter and darker, will work well. Do make sure she's in earshot, or, if she's out of earshot, make sure you have a baby monitor and that it works.

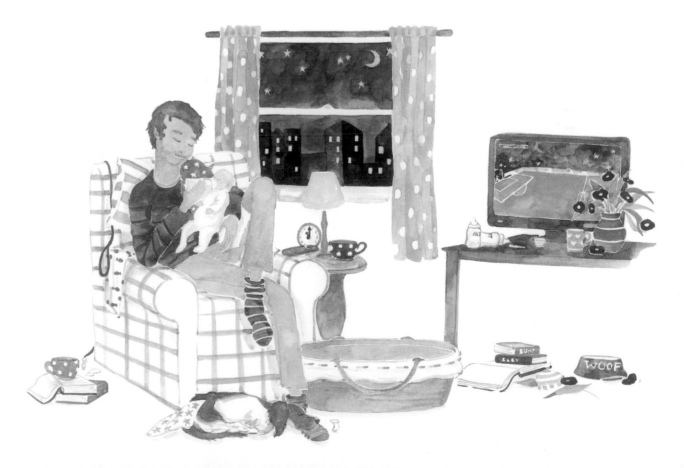

Not quite picture perfect?

Just as you want to take lots of photos of your gorgeous little cherub, be prepared for the fact that she might not be at her most photogenic.

Cradle cap – a slightly scaly, dry, flaky scalp – is very common in babies. It's generally not a problem and often clears up on its own, but mothers find it unattractive. (Try gently washing your baby's hair every day and giving a gentle scrub with your nails or with a soft brush, but avoid picking.)

Your baby might also be suffering from baby acne. This is common in breastfed babies and usually develops in the first few weeks. As unsightly as an outbreak of painful-looking whiteheads are, resist the temptation to squeeze them; they will improve on their own and will not bother your baby.

You might notice that your baby isn't sleeping quite as much; this is fine and to be expected, although it makes your job a little harder. Encourage your baby to enjoy her awake time; maybe put her on a play gym (a mat which has toys hanging from the top) or in a bouncy chair.

By two weeks her umbilical stump should have fallen off, leaving a nice tidy belly button. This might look like a bit of an 'outie' or she may even have a slight hernia. Generally this is nothing to worry about and usually goes in as your baby develops her abdominal muscles.

Hopefully you will have spent the first two weeks resting at home and recovering from the birth, but by three weeks most women are quite keen to start leaving the house. Some new mothers feel like they're only just coping with juggling everything that comes with motherhood and feel that leaving the house would be too much. Do try to get out, even if you're fearful that this might push you over the edge. Humans are naturally sociable beings and being alone in the house with your newborn can be lonely. All women will benefit from adult conversation. As your baby gets older, there are plenty of classes you can do with your baby – baby massage is a great way to catch up with other mums and it's one of the few things your baby will actively enjoy. See page 216 for tips on making your first outing with your baby.

If you're breastfeeding, think about introducing a bottle at this point. This can be of expressed milk, but it's important to make sure your baby is happy feeding from both breast and bottle. If you leave this much later it's much more difficult to introduce. Take the opportunity to leave your partner to do the last feed at night – typically around 10–11pm. Babies will often feed better from the bottle if the person with the breasts isn't giving it to them, and you can get some extra hours' sleep before you're up again in the night.

Although you'll feel a tremendous amount better than you did two weeks ago, remember that you're still recovering and not supposed to be exercising (more than being active) until six weeks after the birth. You should, however, be doing your pelvic floor exercises and try to start engaging your abdominal muscles. Every time you lift something or get up try to pull your tummy in as much as you can – this will do you a lot of good (see pages 232 and 233).

Q&A

'When will I start getting my period again?'
This varies from woman to woman and is often longer for women who have breastfed for longer. If you haven't breastfed at all, your period will probably have returned by three months and some women don't get a period as long as they are breastfeeding. If you're worried you should speak to your GP about it.

Please note: don't think that if you haven't had a period you can't get pregnant; it's less likely but still possible.

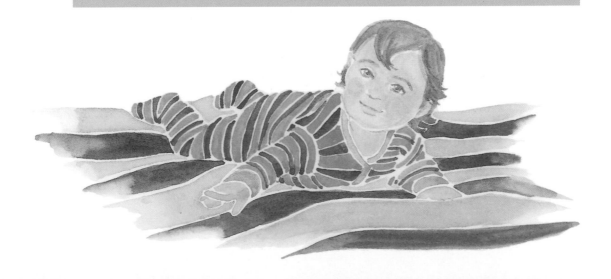

67 Becoming a father:
Caring for mother and baby

Becoming a father will change you; you'll drive home from the hospital more carefully than you've ever driven before, happily ignoring the frustration of the drivers behind you as you navigate the road at 10 mph. You're bringing the most precious thing you have home but suddenly realise it comes with no operating instructions. Don't worry, it's a steep learning curve and, if you get involved, you'll soon become an expert. This chapter will give you an introduction into how to do this, but do also read the postnatal chapters in this book; it will stand you in good stead.

 ## The first few days when mother and baby come home

- Try to get your partner to rest – this is key to her recovery. A generation ago, women would spend a week in hospital after a straightforward delivery. The only reason this is no longer the case is due to cost issues. Encourage her to get into her pyjamas and be in 'recovery mode' for at least three to six days. Your partner will need encouraging and reminding that she needs to take it easy; this is your job.
- A two-hour sleep in the middle of the day is crucial in terms of her recovery, as well as sustaining her while she's up in the night. Even if she doesn't feel like having a sleep, try to persuade her. She's likely to have an emotional crash later on in the day if she doesn't, so be firm.
- Try to do as much for her at home as possible or even persuade a willing friend or mum to help with the cooking, clearing up, washing, cleaning, etc. If you can allow her just to focus on the baby, it will help her enormously.
- Police the visitors; well-meaning friends and relatives are always keen to meet a new baby but they don't always appreciate how inconvenient this might be. Make sure visitors come at a time of day that's convenient for her and make sure they don't stay too long. Try to space them out so they don't all come in the first three days. In a few weeks she will be delighted to have some adult interaction.

Practical things for you to do in the first days

Looking after a newborn baby is all-consuming. If you can organise the bureaucratic part of having a baby, you'll earn serious brownie points ....

- **Register the birth.** A parent needs to register the baby's birth within 42 days. The hospital will give you information about where and when you need to do this and will give you the documentation you'll need.

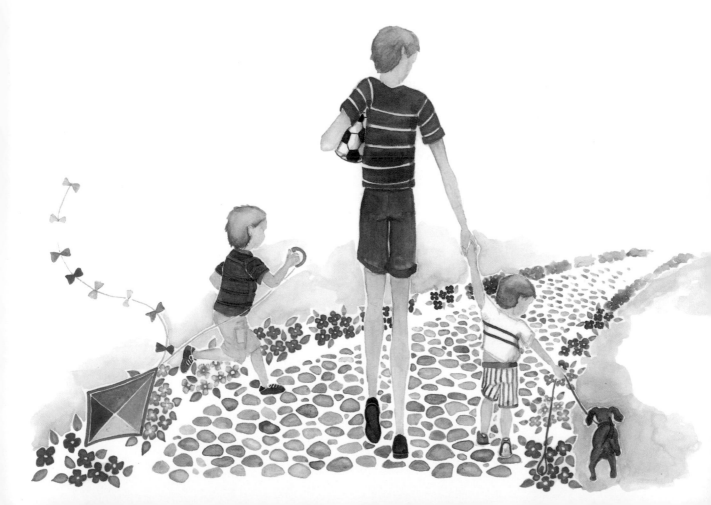

- **Apply for your baby's passport.** You can only do this once the birth has been registered as you'll need to show the birth certificate. Although there is no definite time in which you need to do this, your baby needs to have her own passport to travel, and it can take some time and planning.
- **Health insurance.** If you have health insurance, it's worth adding your baby to it as early as possible.

The baby blues
Due to the massive hormonal changes going on in her body around the time her milk comes in, your partner will probably have a few slightly wobbly days. The baby blues affect some women more than others, but most women do have them. Many women feel a little teary and vulnerable, usually around days three to five. Little things like a cup of spilt tea can set things off and, even if she's not crying, she'll definitely be more sensitive, so be gentle. Support and reassure her; she should return to normal after a few days.

 ## The first weeks with your baby at home
- Try to be hands-on with your baby right from the very beginning. You might be horrified at the prospect of changing your baby's nappy, but in all honesty it's not that bad – and we think every hands-on father will back us up here. Newborn babies' poos are really inoffensive – they actually smell quite nice, and changing your own baby's nappy is usually a great way to interact with her.
- Spend as much time holding your baby as you can. This is all the stimulation she needs in these early days. Don't feel silly talking to her. She will love hearing the sound and tone of your voice and, before you know it, will understand more than you realise.
- If your baby is being breastfed, try to help out with the burping and settling as much as you can (see page 194). It will give your partner a well-earned rest and all this time getting to know your baby will pay off handsomely. If your baby is being fed by bottle, try to get involved with feeds, especially the last feed of the day, usually around 10–11pm. Insist that your partner goes to bed – this is one of the best things you can do – allow her to bank a few precious hours of sleep before she wakes to feed again in the night.
- Immediately after your partner gives birth, she will look about six months pregnant. This is because her uterus, which has grown to accommodate her

baby, takes time to go down. By the time your baby is seven days old, she will probably no longer look visibly pregnant with clothes on, but it will certainly be a while before her body is what it was. Be supportive but remind her that it took nine months for her body to get to term and it's not unreasonable to allow another nine months for it to get back to normal.

● Try to discourage her from doing any major exercise in the first six weeks but thereafter it's a really good idea for her to start building up her core strength again. Apart from making her feel better, she needs to be in good shape to deal with the physical demands of an increasingly mobile baby.

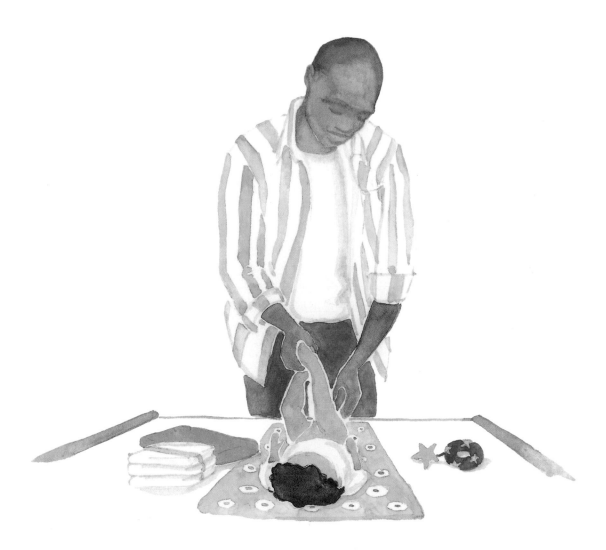

'Nappy changing must be the most overrated fear for new fathers. To be honest, it's not much different to wiping your own bottom – after all, it practically is your own bottom. I actually found changing nappies surprisingly enjoyable. It's one of the few practical things a father can do in the early days and it's all part of the bonding process. It's not nearly as disgusting as fabled; baby poo isn't that bad … until they get on to solids …'
BEN FOGLE

Sex after the baby

You will probably not have sex again after the birth of the baby until at least around six to eight weeks. For around six weeks your partner will bleed as the lining of her uterus sheds. Don't pressurise her to have sex – she will let you know when she is ready. Be prepared; the first few times will not be mind-blowing. You'll probably both be exhausted and she will not be feeling overly confident with the way her body looks, but don't worry: most couples return quickly to an active and enjoyable sex life. If you feel that this is not happening, talk to her about it and encourage her to seek help if necessary.

 ## Postnatal depression

A lot of partners assume that this is very rare; in fact up to 30 per cent of women suffer some degree of postnatal depression, which, if untreated, can continue for years. Women who aren't diagnosed often don't enjoy the first few years of their child's life, so it's really important that it's diagnosed. Partners are often the ones that notice it first.

Read page 179 so you have a good idea of the symptoms of postnatal depression. Do bear in mind that one of the symptoms is an unwillingness of the mother to recognise and talk about postnatal depression. If you feel your partner might be suffering and she denies it, keep monitoring her and, if you are still worried, talk to her GP, midwife or even a family member.

A few general tips for fathers in the first year

● Try to be confident with your baby – she might feel very breakable but as long as you're careful and aware of how to handle her, she will benefit from as much interaction with her father as possible. The more you're involved at this early stage, the more rewarding it will be later on.

- Try to take your baby out to give your partner the chance to really sleep, or simply have some time to herself. Babies will often sleep really well on the go and it's a nice thing to do early on. Your partner will thank you for it (especially if you return with flowers, goodies or food for the fridge). Little things can really lift the mood of an exhausted, overwhelmed and emotional new mother.

- When you take your baby out, get home when you say you will and make sure you have your phone on you. It is not unusual for mothers to be anxious the first time they are not with their babies and panic when they can't get in touch.

- After you go back to work, don't worry if you return to a chaotic house, a crying baby and a teary wife. It will get easier. Just encourage and be supportive. If she's not coping – talk about the idea of getting someone to help. The first months are really tough and tiring but you do turn a corner.

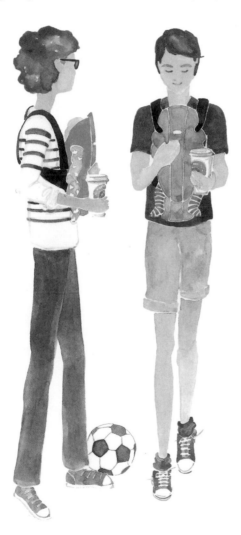

  - Don't forget to nurture your relationship. Don't expect your baby to be the magic glue that will hold your relationship together. If anything, having young children is the stage when it needs most attention. After a few weeks, try to arrange to have dinner just the two of you. Remember, one of the most important things you can give your baby is a strong family unit.

  - Remember that the birth of your baby is exciting but don't expect it to be great fun from day one – newborn babies usually just sleep, feed and cry (some more than others). You will usually only get a smile at six to eight weeks. But put the hours in: it is hugely rewarding when the smiles, laughs and daddy adoration start!

68 The spectrum *of poo*

There is a lot of talk about poo in The Bump Class. We tell the girls that they will all become obsessed about poo – its colour, smell, consistency and regularity, and none of them believe us. By the time we see them at six weeks for the postnatal course they always admit, 'You were right; I didn't believe you, but all we seem to talk about is poo!'

The reason for this is that it's a really good way of seeing whether your baby is being fed enough. In an ideal world our breasts would have little gauges on them which would tell us how much milk our babies had consumed. Sadly this is not the case, and knowing whether your baby has eaten enough is a combination of instinct, feeling how full your breasts are, monitoring weight gain and keeping an eye on what is coming out the other end. A well-fed baby's poo will change colour dramatically in the first two weeks of life, and this colour change is an indication that she is drinking enough. When your health visitor sees you they will always ask about the colour of your baby's poos.

Q&A

'How often should my baby poo?'

How often a baby poos is of huge concern to new mothers, often because, after days of no bowel action, mothers start to fear a 'poonami'. Unfortunately the spectrum of what is normal is very broad. Anywhere from seven times a day to once in seven days is considered normal for breastfed babies.

If you're worried that your baby might be constipated, make sure she's hydrated. There's no need to give her additional water – her milk feeds should be sufficient to hydrate her unless it's unusually hot. However, you could try giving her a little diluted prune juice in her bottle and, if you're really desperate, try lubricating her anus with a little Vaseline on a cotton bud, as this can sometimes ease the delivery.

Baby's poos are not solid and formed like an adult. While just on milk, they will be fairly runny, making leakages common. If your baby's poos are very pale or chalky, especially if she has jaundice, you should seek urgent medical advice.

TIP
If you're concerned about the consistency, colour or smell of poo, keep the nappy and show it to your health visitor, midwife or doctor. Stick it in a nappy bag; they will not think you are crazy, we promise!

Day one	Your baby's first poo, meconium, is a black, tar-like poo that is annoyingly difficult to clean up as it's sticky. It doesn't really smell bad, but you might spend some time getting your baby's bottom clean.
Days two to three	You'll gradually notice the meconium lighten and turn a greeny yellow.
Days four to six	Your baby's poos should be becoming more yellowy. The good news is that it's much easier to clean than the meconium and its smell continues to be inoffensive. It's oddly quite a nice smell – possibly nature's way of introducing parents gently to the delights of nappy changing (see page 181).
Days seven to ten	By day 10 your baby's poos should be consistently mustard yellow, and – once yellow – they should stay that way. If your baby's poos are still a greeny colour by day 10, it's an indication that she's not eating enough, and you should try to feed her more – see pages 185–93.

69 Your first outing *with your baby*

Your baby's first outing can be daunting. While it's definitely worth staying at home for most of the first week, resting and recovering, you will probably reach a stage when you'll get cabin fever and will need to get out. Alternatively you may feel like you're only just coping, and if you do anything to rock the boat, you'll lose the plot. However, this will not happen. You're more likely to lose the plot if you stay holed up at home.

That said, preparing for the first outing often feels like packing for a six-month holiday. The idea of forgetting something will seem like the end of the world, and with babies one tends to pack for every scenario.

Packing list (yes, really!)
- Spare set(s) of clothes (by now you'll know the dangers of the 'poonami')
- Nappies
- Nappy-rash cream
- Nappy bags (plenty of them)
- Wipes
- 2 muslins
- Sterilising wipes
- Hand gel
- Dummies (bring a spare)
- If you're bottle-feeding: bottles, formula, boiled water
- A bib
- If you're breastfeeding: nipple shields, scarf (for modesty when breastfeeding in public)
- Car seat or buggy (or both)
- Spare breast pads
- Nipple cream, if you're using it
- Maternity pads

What you will probably not need:
- A cot (the baby will be able to nap in her car seat or buggy)
- First-aid book
- Shoes for your baby (she's not walking, so there's no point)
- Toys

> 'Whenever I go out now without my baby I take the smallest possible bag – enough to hold a phone, key and credit card. The freedom of not having to lug a small suitcase with me on leaving the house is so liberating!'
> *ALEX, THE BUMP CLASS*

It is common for mothers to feel anxious at the idea of taking their baby out for the day. These are often women who, before their baby arrived, enjoyed successful careers where they were in control of all aspects of their day. Suddenly everything is an unknown; they have had no training in 'baby outings' and the thought of not knowing exactly how the day will pan out can send many intelligent, sensible women into a flurry of panic. If you feel like this, remember that you are not alone; most mothers will have had these anxieties at some point.

The second and subsequent outings are infinitely less stressful. You can cut down on the 'baby paraphernalia' as the baby gets older and there will come a time where you will be able to pop a changing pack and some snacks in your handbag and head out of the door with your little one!

 ## Top tips for a stress-free first outing

- Be organised and plan what you are going to need.
- Don't try to be a superwoman. A short manageable outing is probably a better idea than trying to head out for the whole day.
- Don't plan to do too much on that first outing. One 'task' is probably enough. A trip to the post office, an outing to the shop or a coffee with a friend – but not all three.
- Go out after your baby has had a good feed – feeding in public is probably best left to a later outing.
- Don't go too far from home. It is comforting to know that, if it all kicks off, home is not far away.

 ## When is it safe to take my baby out?

As long as your baby is term and you are feeling up to it, there is no reason not to take your baby out for some fresh air at a few days old. Most people find that they are ready for a more substantial first outing at around two weeks. For the first eight weeks it is advisable to avoid crowded places where the baby may pick up illnesses. Similarly try to discourage too many people and especially strangers from touching the baby in this time. Although your baby's immune system is capable of fighting infections at a young age, the illnesses tend to be more severe, the younger the baby is.

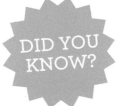
DID YOU KNOW?

A baby's immune system is not fully developed until she is six months old. Until this time she is protected by the antibodies transferred from her mother, both from the placenta and through breastfeeding.

Remember, it is absolutely reasonable to ask visitors to wash their hands or use sterilising gel before touching your baby.

'I was amazed how many well-meaning strangers wanted to stroke my baby's head or cheek when we were out and about. I wasn't comfortable with this as he was so young, so rather than always asking them not to, I took to covering my baby's pram with a blanket. They couldn't see him so didn't want to touch him. Problem solved!' **KARIMA, BUMP CLASS**

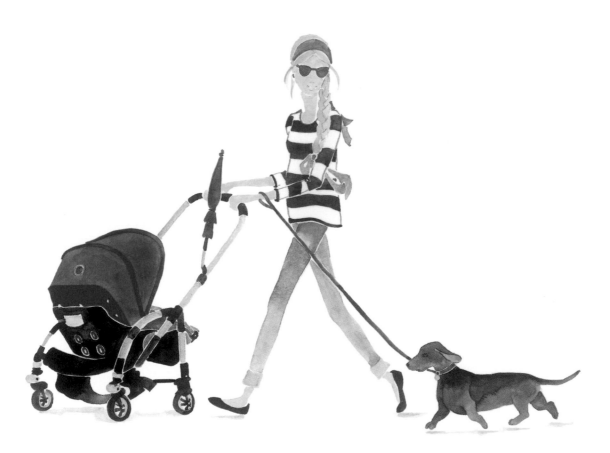

70 Dressing *your baby*

Shopping for your baby is one of the few really fun parts of pregnancy. There are so many adorable little outfits with dinky shoes and tiny colour coordinated socks that are simply irresistible ... but totally impractical. Newborn babies generally hate having their nappies changed – so trying to tie up tiny laces on a pair of designer baby trainers will be a joy you will experience once and never again.

 ## Practical essentials

Baby grows: After their first foray into baby fashion, most mothers prefer to stick to the well-loved and practical baby grow and, for most babies, this is the item of clothing they live in. Ideally they should be 100 per cent cotton and a simple block colour, so that you can wash them on a high cycle if a 'poonami' occurs. Buy them in multipacks and make sure they have feet (trying to keep socks on a newborn is nigh on impossible and if they don't fall off they are certain to get lost in the wash) and ideally scratch mitts too. New babies have long nails that they tend to scratch their faces with. It's not always possible to keep tiny nails perfectly trimmed (see page 184) so it's a good idea in the first weeks to cover their hands with scratch mitts. Some baby grows have these built in, and it just makes life easier having it all incorporated.

When choosing your baby grows, don't worry about the detail on their collars. What will become crucial to you is how easily they can be done up. Some fancy ones have complicated back openings or, even worse, miniature buttons that you will have to negotiate every time you change your baby's outfit. Bearing in mind this can happen several times an hour, easy access is essential. Poppers down the front are fail-safe.

Nightgowns: Many mothers like putting their babies in nightgowns at night. These are essentially the same as a baby grow on the top but, instead of having legs, they have an elasticated opening below the feet, making swift night-time nappy changes mercifully easy.

Vests: Depending on the season, you'll need some vests – either long-sleeved or short-sleeved – to go under the baby grow. Make sure these have poppers at the bottom. As you're constantly lifting your baby, anything that is not fastened below the groin will ride up and become uncomfortable.

Cardigans: For when it's a little colder, it's worth having a couple of cardigans. Thin cardigans are better than thick bulky ones.

Hats: These are essential, and your baby should wear one every time she goes outside, unless it is particularly hot. In the summer cotton hats will suffice, but for the winter woollen ones are better.

Outdoor suit: For winter babies an outdoor suit is really useful as it avoids multiple layers of clothing. This should have feet, gloves and a hood. Make sure it's appropriate for the temperature of where you live.

A few general rules when buying clothes for your baby

Sizing is confusing. Most newborn babies will be in the newborn size (NB) but they will outgrow this in a few weeks so it's worth getting everything in the next size up, 0–3 months, instead. Some brands do sizes for premature babies (John Lewis are good), but sizes also tend to differ among labels. As a generalisation, the more upmarket the brand, the smaller the size, and the French ones are the worst. French babies appear to be very small indeed.

'My husband lovingly bought our son an outdoor suit from Toronto, where the temperature drops to -30°C. In spite of it being "the coldest winter for 20 years" it was never quite cold enough for our son to wear this suit. The most important thing to consider is how easy it is to get your baby in and out.'
MARINA

Make sure you don't overdress your baby. It's something we see so frequently and it's potentially very dangerous for your baby, who finds it difficult to regulate her temperature. Babies should never have hats on indoors and the ideal room temperature for a baby is 18°C (64°F). Generally babies should be wearing one extra layer than you are. If you're unsure, feel the back of her neck, which will give you a good indication of whether she's too hot.

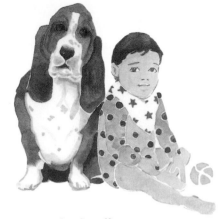

 ## Washing your baby's clothes

Be realistic about caring for your baby's clothes. Motherhood has enough challenges without having to hand-wash your baby's clothes.

People are often concerned about which detergents they should use for their baby. Our advice is not to change what you are using unless your baby develops any kind of skin complaint. The most important thing is that your baby's clothes are washed well and that anything with faeces on is soaked in an antibacterial soak before washing.

TIP

In spite of the modern technology dedicated to developing nappies, poo invariably escapes. The best way to get any kind of stain out is to soak it in cold water with antibacterial soak and then put it on a long, cold wash. Hot water tends to cement the stain, making it impossible to get out. This tends to work for all stains, from carrot purée to squashed strawberries.

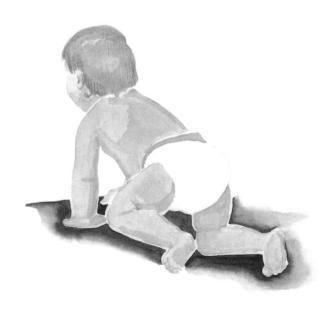

71 You and your *baby at six weeks*

Six weeks is a big milestone as far as your baby is concerned. By now she will be a lot more awake and will be taking in her surroundings with interest. She will begin to communicate with you through her looks, her noises and her facial expressions. You should get your first smile by this stage, and before you know it she will be cooing and giggling and loving interaction. It is a great reward for all your effort.

Talk to your baby as much as you can. Although she doesn't yet understand the words you are using, she will be learning basic communication skills. It is also good for your relationship with her if you treat her as a little person right from the beginning rather than 'just a baby'.

Six weeks is also a big milestone for you, and it's the time many mothers describe as finally feeling more human again. You will probably have developed a routine with your baby and will be beginning to understand her. Some lucky mothers will be getting a bit more sleep, with some babies sleeping for six- or seven- hour stints during the night, but many babies will only be managing four hours at a time. Even mothers of the best sleepers will probably still feel sleep-deprived, but the fog will be lifting. Feeding should be well established and you will probably be confident enough to be feeding out and about. Hopefully you will have begun to plan or develop a bit of a social life with your baby, meeting other friends with babies and enjoying outings.

The six-week check

You and your baby will have a check-up with your GP some time between six and eight weeks. You should bring your baby's red book (which will have been given to you when you left hospital or by your health visitor). Make sure you use this opportunity to discuss any concerns you may have about your baby, such as colic, reflux, rashes, feeding and sleep.

Your baby
- The doctor will check your baby's weight and perhaps her length and head circumference.
- They will also do a full physical examination from head to toe, including fontanelles, eyes, ears, mouth, heart and lungs, abdominal organs, genitals, hips (to check for alignment and stability) and reflexes.

- The doctor will ask you about your baby's development, feeding and sleeping patterns and bowel movements. You will also discuss vaccinations, which start at eight weeks (see page 241).

You

This check is about you as much as your baby. The doctor will want to know about the birth and how well you have recovered. They will ask you questions about how you are coping emotionally with motherhood and look for signs of postnatal depression. They will also do the following checks:

- Your blood pressure and urine will be checked and your doctor may weigh you and give you advice on getting back to exercise.
- Your tummy will be felt to check the uterus has shrunk back down to its original size (about the size of an apple), and you will be asked about any continued bleeding. You should be prepared for them to do an internal examination if necessary.
- If you have had a caesarean your scar will be checked.
- If you have stitches down below they may check those too, although they will have dissolved by now. If you want the area checked and they don't offer, ask them.
- Most doctors will ask about feeding and check your breasts and nipples if necessary.
- Your doctor will ask about whether you have returned to sex and will want to discuss contraception. (Remember, breastfeeding is not a reliable form of contraception – you can get pregnant very soon after giving birth.) If you opt to use a coil for contraception, this can be fitted at this time.
- If you are due a smear it can be done at the six-week check.

Q&A

'Is incontinence or leakage after birth normal – and will it stop?'
It's normal to experience a little bit of incontinence after you've given birth, which is why we're constantly banging on about doing your pelvic floor exercises. If you've been doing these (see page 44), you should have strengthened your pelvic floor sufficiently by six weeks for you not to experience any leakage, but if you are, it's important to discuss this with your GP. They might refer you to a women's health physiotherapist, who should be able to resolve any problems. Try not to be embarrassed about this; it's only going to get better if you do something about it. Remember, it's usually something that is very easily fixed.

Sex

Getting back to sex after having a baby is the last thing on most girls' minds. As well as being exhausted, you'll probably not feel great about your body. Some women feel a little worried about how it's going to feel, especially after a vaginal delivery. You might want to think about sex again around the six-week mark. When you do feel ready, the first time probably won't be mind-blowing, but it shouldn't be consistently painful and will get much more enjoyable.

'After my baby was born, sex was the last thing I felt like, but I was worried that if we put it off for too long it might become an issue. With my leaky breasts and wobbly tummy it turned about to be more funny than passionate, but actually it got swiftly better from there ... and I'm now pregnant again.' JENNY, THE BUMP CLASS'

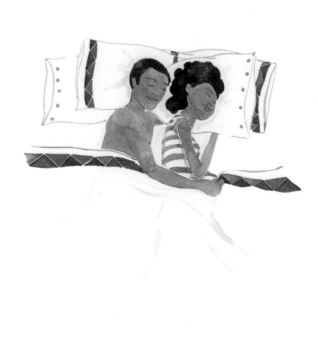

Options for contraception postnatally

Mini-pill (progesterone-only pill): This is a type of pill you can use when you are breastfeeding. It works well but you have a narrower window to take it compared to the normal combined contraceptive pill.

Progesterone-only implants or injection.

Coil: Some women who have coils fitted before they've given birth find putting one in very painful. After birth most mothers find this process painless and the coil a brilliant form of contraception. As and when you would like to think about having another baby, it's quickly taken out and your fertility returns to normal. There are two types of coil:

- **The copper coil (or IUD)** makes the uterus inhospitable for sperm and eggs to survive and also stops a fertilised egg implanting in the womb. It does not use any hormones but can make periods heavier and more painful.

- **The hormone coil (or IUS)** releases a small amount of hormone locally into the uterus. This acts as a contraceptive by making it difficult for sperm to move through the cervix and by thickening the lining of the womb so that it can't accept a fertilised egg. In some cases the hormone also stops ovulation. It is very popular with women postnatally as periods become much lighter and often stop altogether.

Barrier methods (condoms/femidoms): As long as you remember and use them properly, these are a good contraceptive.

Natural methods: Some people prefer to just monitor the body for signs of ovulation. This method is not very reliable. You need to be very organised about doing it at the same time every day.

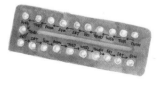
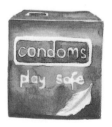

72 Your baby's sleep in *the first months*

In the first few months, babies don't do much more than sleep and feed. As you'll soon realise, life becomes all about the sleep. If they've slept well, babies tend to be happier when they're awake and feed better. Amazingly, babies who have had good sleeps during the day, tend to sleep better at night.

In the early days your baby should be with you the whole time – around the house in the days and with you in the bedroom at night. It is a good option to have her in a Moses basket, as these are light and easy to move to wherever you are. Once you're finding that your baby's sleep is being disrupted by noise and light, you might want to start thinking about moving her into her own space to sleep. As soon as she's not within earshot, you should have a baby monitor.

Swaddling

Most babies love being swaddled. They've spent nine months confined to your uterus and a lot of babies like the security of being confined into a swaddle. Babies are also born with a reflex called the 'Moro reflex'; this makes their arms fly out to the sides, often about 30 minutes after they've gone to sleep, waking them up. Swaddling stops this happening.

How to swaddle your baby
You can use any large piece of cloth as long as it is not too thick, is breathable and has some sort of 'give' to it.
- Place the cloth on the floor and fold the top corner down.
- Place your baby's shoulders just below the folded edge.
- Fold one side tightly over that arm and tuck it under the body on the opposite side.
- Fold up the bottom corner over the feet.
- Tightly wrap the remaining side over the whole baby, tucking the edge under the baby.
- You should ensure the swaddle is tight on her arms but looser on her bottom half, allowing her legs to bend up and out at the hips, in a 'frog' position.

Most parents swaddle their babies too loosely and the baby ends up wriggling out and waking herself up by flinging her arms around. As long as the material has 'give' it is very hard to do it too tightly.

226

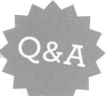

'Will swaddling cause my baby to have hip problems?'
Studies have linked traditional swaddling – where the baby's legs are tightly bound, extended, together and straight out – to hip dysplasia. It is, however, safe to swaddle your baby as long as the swaddle is looser on her bottom half, allowing her legs to bend up and out at the hips, in a 'frog' position, as directed above.

 ## Getting your baby to sleep
Babies like being rocked to sleep, and in the early days there is no problem with this. As your baby approaches four to six weeks though, it's a good idea if she starts to learn to go to sleep on her own. Try to put her down in her cot awake so that she learns to do this. Some babies are soothed by music or white noise, which is fine as you can just switch it on and leave. What you want to avoid in the long run is your baby becoming dependent on something that only you can do in order to get her to sleep.

 ## Dummies
Dummies are often regarded as the ultimate evil, particularly by older generations. In our view, a dummy used purely for sleep can really help soothe sucky babies. What you want to avoid at all costs is your child running around aged two with a dummy constantly in her mouth.

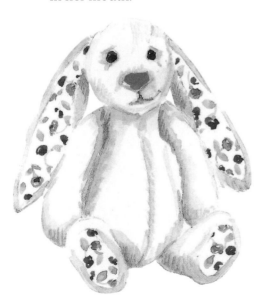

If you are going to use a dummy we advise:
- Take a dummy with you to hospital – a lot of new parents soothe their newborns with their little finger in their mouths. It's much easier (and more hygienic) to use a dummy.
- Very quickly establish that you only use the dummy for sleep. A good rule is to only keep it in the cot. If a dummy is only used for sleep it won't interfere with language development or teeth.

Babies often start waking once they spit their dummies out, and parents say that they go in up to 20 times a night to put it back in. This is terrible for both the mother and baby, and if this is happening we advise that you take the dummy away immediately.

Taking the dummy away
Either do this before six months or, once you can reason with them, at around two–three years old. In between it's a hard thing to give up and they are too young to understand why.

- Once you've decided to take the dummy away, actually throw away every dummy in the house. If you've just put them in a drawer, it will be too tempting to give in and give one back.
- Be prepared for a bit of crying but be strong; this phase will be relatively short. A lot of Bump Class girls expect the 'cold turkey' approach in removing the dummy to be hell, but actually are very surprised how easily their baby forgets about it.
- Don't give in – if you do, it will negate all your hard work up to this point.

 ## Safety guidelines for avoiding cot death
Cot death is every parent's worst fear, and we want to do everything we can to prevent it. Thankfully today, it is very rare indeed and, as long as you're following the basic guidelines below, it's not something you should be worrying about.

Below are guidelines for what we know we can do to reduce the risk:

- Put your baby to sleep on her back. Since the 'Back to Sleep' campaign was introduced in the 1990s, advising parents that it is safer to put babies to sleep on their backs, the incidence of cot death has decreased by over 50 per cent.
- Do not allow anyone to smoke in the house. Smoking in pregnancy increases the risk of cot death by 40 per cent, and smoking in the house where the baby lives increases the risk by 80 per cent. If you have a family member who resents not being allowed to smoke in your house, don't be afraid to quote these statistics.
- Don't let your baby overheat. Too cold is better than too hot.
- Do not sleep with your baby in your bed with you. If you want to co-sleep, use a co-sleeping cot, which latches onto the side of your bed, giving your baby her own space and protecting her.
- Don't fall asleep on a sofa or chair while holding your baby.

- Always put your baby's feet at the bottom of her cot or Moses basket, so if she wriggles, she wriggles upwards.
- Breastfeeding is protective. Although we don't know exactly why, studies have shown that breastfed babies are at lower risk of cot death.
- Once out of the swaddle, sleeping bags as opposed to blankets are considered to be safer because babies can not wriggle underneath them.

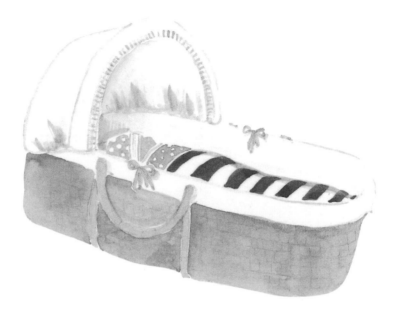

'My mother was adamant that, since she had always put her children to sleep on their fronts and we all survived, it was perfectly safe for me to do the same with my baby. It was really useful to have discussed this on The Bump Class and be able to give her the powerful statistics.'
LOUISA, THE BUMP CLASS

73 Mothers' *sleep*

Sleep might once have been something you took for granted, but once you're a mother every minute you can get is precious. The key to enjoying motherhood is making sure you are getting as much sleep as you can – if necessary even changing your entire attitude to sleep. Continued sleep deprivation will have a cumulative effect on your mood, sanity and ability as a mother. It makes you weak, short-tempered and ill-prepared to deal with the trials of motherhood.

Rules of sleep as a mother

1. Until your baby is sleeping through the night you should be having a nap in the middle of the day. An hour in bed will give you the energy you need to enjoy your baby.
2. Try to avoid going to bed late. Mothers are great procrastinators; it's easy to be distracted by other chores and find yourself going to bed at midnight. Try setting an alarm at 9pm or 10pm to ensure you get to bed at a sensible hour.
3. You need to learn to prioritise sleep. If you have to cancel dinners, or if your house is not as spotless as it used to be, so be it. Your job as a mother is the most crucial one and your ability to do it well depends on you getting enough sleep.

As the opportunity to sleep becomes rarer, you need to maximise the sleep you are getting. Mothers are frequently woken by their children and many, once woken, take too long to get back to sleep again. Efficient sleep makes motherhood significantly easier so if you can go straight back to sleep, rather than waste an hour tossing and turning, you'll cope better.

Refer back to the list of suggestions on page 85 for helping you sleep during your pregnancy. You'll find these techniques are just as useful now you are a new mother. You can try implementing some of the methods that worked before, but it's also worth trying different ones; you might find you now can't get to sleep for very different reasons. Remember that if you use any white noise, music or radio to aid your sleep, you should always make sure you can still hear your baby if she cries.

'Every mother will tell you that the hardest thing to cope with is sleep deprivation. It is after all a torture technique. That said, if you've had a terrible night, resist the temptation to waste emotional energy worrying about how you're going to get through the day. The reality is that you can exist on less sleep than you thought. For me this realisation came when my second child was born. The night before my nephew's christening, Iona didn't sleep for one minute, until 6:30am, 15 minutes before her brother woke up. Deranged with fatigue, my husband and I knocked back a dangerous amount of coffee and drove to the country, not understanding how we could possibly survive a day of socialising while looking after our children. But it was actually great fun. A rare, glorious summer's day, Iona slept while Ludo played in the garden, and aided by a glass of wine, we relished the first opportunity to have an interesting conversation, our first emergence from the two-children-under-two fog. Remember the fear of severe fatigue is often far worse than the reality, so try not to think about it too much, and just get on with it.' *MARINA*

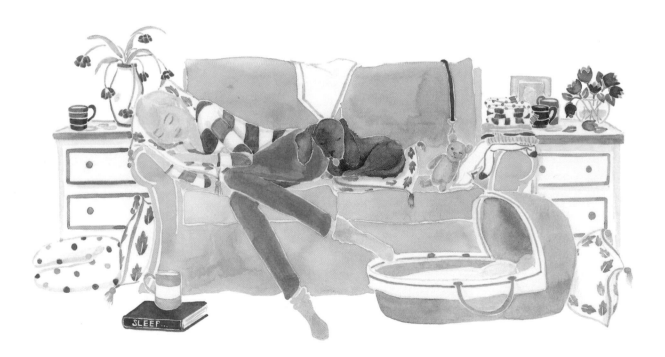

74 Postnatal *exercise*

 ## Immediately post birth

The most important exercises to be doing immediately after birth are your pelvic floor exercises. These are exactly the same as those you were doing in pregnancy – see page 44. Initially you might not feel like a whole lot is going on down there while you're doing them in the few days after birth, but it's important to keep going and you'll soon feel the difference.

Strengthening your core is also important after you've had a baby. By the end of your pregnancy the main muscles that run down the front of your abdomen have stretched and, in many cases, have separated down the midline (known as diastasis recti). While this is normal in pregnancy, it's important that you work on gradually retraining and strengthening them once your baby is born. These core muscles are crucial in supporting your back and pelvis and, as your baby gets heavier, you'll need them to be strong and working effectively to care for her.

Sit-ups aren't going to do anything but damage initially, but what you can do in the early days is try to remember to engage (gently draw in) your tummy and pelvic floor muscles every time you lift something, bend down or lean over the changing table. After a few days of doing this, it will become second nature and if you can do this without thinking, your body will thank you.

'After my first pregnancy, I don't think I ever really thought about strengthening my core and I paid for it during my second pregnancy, which was dominated by back pain. After my second child was born, I really tried to focus on gently pulling my lower tummy muscles in constantly but there was so much to do that it was quite easy to forget. Then my physio told me to wear an 'inappropriately tight' top when I was in the house on my own. It was perfect and made me subconsciously always engage those weakened abs.' MARINA

Walking is a great way to ease your body gently back into a bit of cardiovascular exercise and you can do it with your baby. Don't make that first walk a two-hour power walk, but it's something you can gradually build up to.

Bump Class girls often ask how effective corsets or belly bands are in getting your waist back post pregnancy. The idea behind most of these bands is that they support the weakened abdominal muscles and reduce any further bulging or straining, particularly with activities such as lifting, sneezing or sitting up. But in order to get your waist back and tummy flat you also need to strengthen your stomach muscles. So if you're using a corset in conjunction with safe postnatal strengthening exercises, then brilliant, but don't bank on simply wearing a corset daily to ensure your waist gets back to normal.

TIP
Extreme exercise will affect the volume of breast milk you're producing.

Six weeks after birth

Whether you've had a natural birth or caesarean, you should wait until you're given the green light to exercise again at the six-week check with your doctor before you don your gym gear. This is really important advice that you should stick to, however tempting the cross-trainer might seem. The time goes by quickly and you have a real chance of injuring yourself if you start too early.

Once you've had the all-clear to exercise, it's important to take it slowly. This is not the time to go for a 4-mile run around the park. Start with low-intensity and low-impact exercise that really focuses on further strengthening that all-important core (postnatal Pilates, yoga and barre-core classes are all good examples) and gradually build up to the kind of exercise you were doing before you were pregnant.

It's not uncommon for women to experience slight urinary leakage when they first start more intensive exercise, especially running. If this is happening, or if you are worried about an ongoing gap down the centre of your abdominal muscles, see a women's health physiotherapist. Do not ignore these things or they can get worse.

75 Adjusting to life with *Twins or multiples*

Giving birth to twins or multiples is joyous but for many, particularly those who know just how hard looking after one baby can be, the prospect of two can be terrifying. Whatever anyone tells you, bringing up twins is challenging, especially in the early months. Everything is twofold. Twice as many feeds, twice as many nappies, twice as much crying and quite possibly you being twice as sleep-deprived and overwhelmed. But don't forget, without doubt you have twice the smiles, hugs, first steps, giggles and twice the joy. And, of course, your babies will forever have a close friend and a built-in playmate.

 ## Routines

Every mother of twins that we've met agrees that getting twins into the same feeding and sleeping routine is essential. It is very hard to feed twins together, but it is possible and the sooner you master this, the better. If you end up feeding them at different times, there will be no time for anything else and it becomes very easy for exhaustion and low mood to set in.

There is no magic routine for twins, and it is fine to follow the same gentle and flexible routine that you may do for singletons. The key is that they learn to feed, settle and sleep at the same time. Most mothers find that the babies very quickly learn to sleep through each other's crying; however, if yours are light sleepers and you want to keep them in the same room then background 'white noise' can really help.

 ## Feeding

- The key for feeding twins is to have lots of cushions handy. You can buy all sorts of feeding pillows, but most mothers agree that normal pillows do the job just as well. If you're breastfeeding, put a pillow under each of your arms and use the 'rugby ball' hold to feed the babies simultaneously. For bottle-feeding, you can hold each baby in the crook of your arm and hold each bottle with the opposite arm. Another technique is to cradle one and have the other on your knees with your knees up.
- Once they're a little bigger, putting them in identical bouncy chairs (at the same height) is a brilliant way to feed them. Get light, bouncy chairs so that you can pick up a baby that needs to be burped one-handed from the chair. It sounds tricky but it's doable.

THE BUMP CLASS

- Healthy newborn babies of average size need to feed every 3–4 hours. Twins, even at term, are usually slightly smaller than singletons and smaller babies need to be fed nearer the three-hourly mark. It's important to wake them for three-hourly feeds if they're not waking themselves.

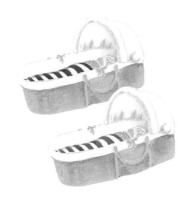

- As with singletons, if you are breastfeeding you should consider offering a bottle of expressed breast milk early on. It's important that the babies get used to feeding from both breast and bottle, in part so that you can share some of the responsibility of feeding but also to give you some flexibility if your milk supply dwindles and your babies need top-ups.

- If you're not managing to produce quite enough breast milk to feed both your babies, consider pumping after each feed; this will stimulate your body to produce more milk. This is time-consuming and exhausting so, if you're going to go down this route, hire a hospital-grade double breast pump and a pumping bra. It's hideous but will enable you to actually use your hands while pumping. Motherhood is all about multi-tasking.

- We all know that breastfeeding is best for your babies, but supplying enough milk for two babies can be difficult for some mothers. If you find you have to top up, don't beat yourself up about it. It's tough enough being a mother to twin babies without feeling guilty about something you can't control.

- If you're planning to breastfeed your twins, you really need to make sure that you're eating healthy, nutritious food to boost your supply, and you will be amazed by how much you consume.

Coping with twice the crying

Mothers of twins all have to get used to the sound of their babies crying. It's not that they're negligent mothers, but that often they're busy with one and simply can't get to the other. Listening to your baby cry is horrid for you as her mother, but remember your baby won't be hurt by crying and you will get to her as soon as you can. If her 'complaint' is minor, chances are she will have stopped by the time you get to her.

Sleep

Twins are often put into the same cot after they're born and this can be comforting for them. Once they start grabbing things (like their sibling), it's time to let them have their own space. Start by moving them further apart in the cot; it will make the switch-over easier. There is no hard and fast rule as to when to do this, but most people find it happens at around 12 weeks.

Sleep is essential for your recovery, and it's imperative that you sleep whenever the babies sleep. Don't be too fastidious about the other things that need to be done – sleep should be at the top of your list of priorities (remember the sleep rules on page 230). As soon as your babies are asleep or you have help, switch off your phone and get into bed.

Help

- Help, if you can get it, is key. Try to get your partner as involved and hands-on as early as possible. Most new fathers suffer from a lack of confidence and a mistaken concern that they aren't qualified to look after their babies. Don't let them believe this. The sooner they're confident with the babies, the more they can help. Of course, this is less of an 'option' with twins – most fathers of twins end up mucking in from day one because they have to.
- Try to get your partner to master the art of feeding both at the same time as this will allow you to catch up on precious sleep while they're feeding. Don't waste your resources: if he can feed the babies, let him get on with it so you can do something constructive.
- Do try to allow anyone else to help you – mothers, in-laws, friends, neighbours – even if it is just an hour during the day, taking the babies for a walk in the pram to give you a break. This will give you some time off but also allow you to spend some precious time alone with your partner. Parenthood strains a relationship at the best of times, but with twins, the stresses are double. Having a strong healthy relationship is the best thing you can do for your children.
- Most mothers of twins agree that having support from other mothers of twins is invaluable. It is worth joining a local twins group after the babies are born. Have a look at the Tamba (Twins and Multiple Births Association) website for details of a group local to you: www.tamba.org.uk/clubs

Baths

Bath time is tricky and it is really important to have help. It's not safe to bath twins together on your own, even in bath seats, until they're really good at sitting up. If you're on your own you will have to bath them one at a time.

Relaxation

It is stressful being a mother of twins but being stressed is only going to hinder your ability to cope as a mother. Try to make time for something that helps you to relax. Just because you've given birth, don't forget any hypnotherapy or relaxation techniques that you learnt in advance of your birth. Yoga and meditation can also really help mothers relax in the precious time available to them. If that is not for you, go for a walk, watch a film or do some cooking – whatever relaxes you is good in the long run.

Don't worry about your ability to cope long term and please don't try to do everything perfectly. For every parent – of a singleton or of twins – perfection is nigh on impossible; good enough is all you need to be. At the end of the day the most important thing is that you have fun and establish a loving and nurturing relationship with your babies.

Yes, it's a challenge but, as challenges go, bringing up twins is possibly one of the most rewarding.

'Because twins have to learn to share and wait their turn from day one, they often become laid-back characters. Once they start interacting they actually become easier as they entertain each other. There is nothing quite like watching your twins giggling with each other. It is amazing!'
MARY, THE BUMP CLASS

76 Red flags for you and your *baby in the first month*

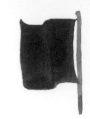

When you become a mother (or father) you develop what is known as 'parental instinct'. You probably won't realise that you have it until you use it. It is extremely powerful and not to be ignored. Doctors are trained to take parents seriously even if they can't put their finger on what is wrong. No good doctor or nurse will berate you for unnecessarily taking your baby to be checked over if you feel she is not right.

We can't cover all emergency scenarios in detail in this book but we advise all new parents and carers to do a paediatric first-aid course to give them confidence and prepare them for an emergency.

Rule number one – trust your instinct.

When to speak to a doctor about your baby
If your baby has:
- A temperature or fever (over 37.5°C/99.5°F for a newborn)
- Worsening jaundice, especially if combined with pale stools and dark urine
- A rash and is unwell. Babies tend to get rashes, most of which are skin complaints and are not an emergency. If your baby has a rash and is unwell with it she should be seen by a doctor
- Breathing difficulties of any sort
- Blood from anywhere
- Persistent vomiting and diarrhoea – your baby probably has a bug, but can get dehydrated very quickly so seek medical advice
- Projectile vomiting – this is usually very dramatic
- A change in cry – particularly if it becomes more feeble or weak than usual (you will get to know your baby's cries very well and will know when it changes)
- Serious problems settling and cries persistently, especially if combined with a fever
- Become limp or floppy, or very sleepy, is not waking for feeds and not feeding well once woken
- A convulsion or anything that could have been a convulsion

> *'Trust your instinct; parents know their babies best, and if they feel something is "not quite right" they are usually correct.'*
> YIANNIS IOANNOU, CONSULTANT PAEDIATRICIAN

When to speak to a doctor about yourself

There are certain medical problems that you are more at risk of in the days and weeks following childbirth. You should call a doctor if you suffer from any of the following:

- Fever or pain in the tummy or back
- Shortness of breath or chest pain
- Lots of large clots in your vaginal bleeding
- A swollen leg on one side
- Mastitis (see box)
- Change in bleeding, such as smelly discharge
- Mood changes (see postnatal depression on page 179)
- Redness around your caesarean scar (this could be a wound infection)
- Consistently painful sex
- Worsening abdominal pain

Mastitis

This is an infection of the breast tissue usually triggered by a blocked milk duct. It affects 1 in 10 women in the first three months of breastfeeding. It ranges from early mastitis – usually a tender area on the breast – to full-blown mastitis, which is particularly nasty.

Thankfully there are warning signs, and it's really important that these are on your radar. That way you can see a doctor and be treated – and hopefully avoid a nasty case of mastitis.

Warning signs:
- Tender and red area on breast
- Little lump
- Harder patches on your breast

As soon as you feel any of the above, you should:
- Continue to breastfeed from both breasts as normal.
- Make sure your baby is latching properly.
- Gently massage any hard areas where milk isn't draining from down towards the nipple to help drain any blocked ducts.
- Massage your breasts from the top when you're in the shower to relieve any blockages, and use the hot water to relieve any tenderness.
- Drink plenty of water.
- Wear loose-fitting clothing and a well-fitting nursing bra (not underwired).
- Take painkillers (anything the hospital has given you postnatally will not affect breastfeeding).

You should see your GP as soon as possible if, in spite of these measures, you feel it's getting worse, or any of the following symptoms start developing:
- Increasing red patches of skin, which are getting hotter and more tender
- An enlarging tender lump or area of hardness under the skin
- Nipple discharge, which can be bloody
- Burning breast pain – either continuously or while breastfeeding

Full-on mastitis will make you feel very unwell – as though you've got a nasty flu with a high fever, all-over body ache and no energy. To avoid this happening, it's crucial that you don't delay seeing your GP. Mastitis is usually easily treated with antibiotics that will not affect your breastfeeding.

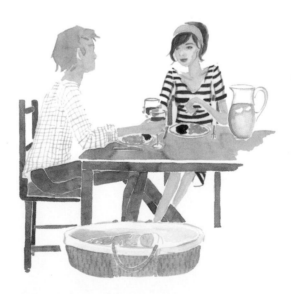

77 Vaccinations

Vaccinations have saved the lives of millions of children. Because these vaccines are given worldwide with virtually no negative consequences, the medical world agrees that they are incredibly safe. In fact, choosing not to vaccinate your child would be considered irresponsible; these vaccinations protect against illnesses that, if your child contracts, could kill or seriously harm them. Vaccination also prevents the spread of disease among the vulnerable. If your child contracts an illness that could have been prevented by vaccination, she risks passing it onto young unvaccinated babies or people who can't be vaccinated.

What vaccinations will my baby have and when?

The current UK vaccination schedule is in the 'red book' given to you shortly after the birth. This does change, which is why we have not included it here. Because of the importance of vaccinations, we advise asking your GP if you have any questions about what vaccinations to have when.

Additional vaccinations

It is worth knowing that there are some extra vaccinations you may choose to have which, rather like travel vaccinations, are available privately or at an additional cost through your GP. These are:

- Chickenpox: Routinely given in many countries, this two-dose vaccine protects your child from the chickenpox infection. It can be given from one year.
- BCG: This protects against tuberculosis and is usually given soon after birth but not routinely throughout the UK. If you think your baby is going to travel in her life, it's worth asking if this can be done.
- There are various additional vaccinations that you may want to consider, especially if you might live in other countries. These vary so discuss with your doctor what would be appropriate.

Dispelling vaccine myths

Separating vaccinations provides no benefit; rather it's more traumatic as your baby has to have more injections, so medics group as many as is safe and viable into one jab.

In 1998 a doctor claimed that the MMR (measles, mumps and rubella) vaccine was linked to autism. However, this study has subsequently been entirely discredited. Since then multiple large studies have shown that there is no link between the two. Indeed, the doctor responsible was subsequently struck off the medical register and bears the responsibility for a large number of deaths and permanent injuries as a result of parents not vaccinating their children.

Vaccines cannot overload a child's immune system. From the day she's born, your baby's immune system has to deal with exposure to different bacteria and viruses every day and the immune system is able to cope perfectly well. To put it into perspective, if a child was given 11 vaccinations at the same time it would only use a thousandth of its immune system.

'Vaccinations are one of the most important things I do, but also one of the things I least like doing as I hate seeing a baby distressed. I find that if the baby is feeding while I give the vaccination, they sometimes don't even cry at all. Alternatively, distracting the baby immediately with a rattle or rain maker often means they forget about it in seconds.'
CHIARA

Vaccination tips

- Don't count on your GP reminding you when the next vaccinations are due; put them in your diary.
- Plan a convenient time for the jabs – bearing in mind that your baby might be more grizzly for up to 48 hours after the vaccinations. Choose a time when you've got extra help and support and no plans, rather than the day before her christening or a long-haul flight!
- Don't forget to bring your child's personal health record – the 'red book', which will have been given to you shortly after birth. It's crucial that the vaccinations are recorded.
- Some mothers give their baby some infant paracetamol an hour before her appointment and keep it handy for afterwards. It's quite normal for babies to be more restless, fractious and grumpy and even to develop a mild temperature. The injection site often becomes a bit red and sore. Serious reactions to vaccinations are incredibly rare, but if you're worried, call your GP.
- Remember the injections are not particularly painful for your baby – the cries are more a form of objection and shock rather than pain. Arguably the whole process is far more agonising for the mother!

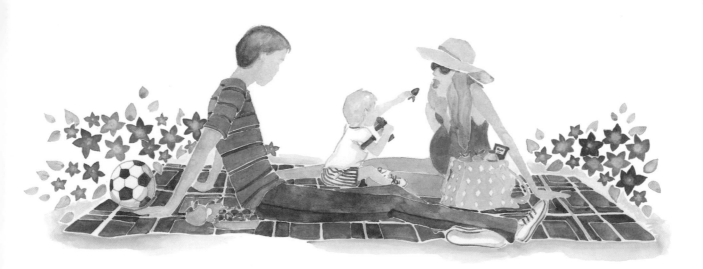

Glossary

active labour/established labour the stage of labour when your cervix dilates from 4–10 cm and contractions come regularly at 3–5-minute intervals. At this stage of birth the mother should go to hospital or be accompanied by a midwife.

acupuncture a system of complementary medicine that involves pricking the skin or tissues with needles, used to alleviate pain and to treat various physical, mental, and emotional conditions. Originating in ancient China, acupuncture is now widely practised in the West.

afterbirth the placenta and fetal membranes discharged from the womb after the birth of the baby.

afterpains caused by the womb contracting back to its pre-pregnancy size. The pains may feel similar to period pains, though sometimes the pain can be severe. It takes weeks, rather than days, for the womb to return to its normal size.

ageing placenta when the placenta is not working well in late pregnancy; labour would usually be induced if this occurs.

amniocentesis a diagnostic test for chromosomal abnormalities such as Down's syndrome, done using a sample of the amniotic fluid. This is usually only offered if there is a high risk that the baby will develop a serious condition or abnormality. It is usually carried out between 15 and 20 weeks of pregnancy.

amniotic fluid the fluid surrounding a fetus in the womb.

amniotic sac a bag of fluid inside the womb where the fetus develops and grows.

anaemia a condition in which the blood cannot carry enough oxygen to meet the needs of the body.

anaesthetic (general) medication that induces a state of controlled unconsciousness, so the recipient is unaware of surgery and doesn't move or feel pain while it is carried out.

anaesthetic (local) medication causing a complete loss of pain sensation to a specific area of the body without loss of consciousness.

anomaly scan the ultrasound scan that occurs around 20 weeks to look closely at how the fetus and her organs are developing.

antenatal relating to pregnancy and the time before birth.

anterior position is where the back of the baby's head is at the front. The majority of babies lie this way.

apgar score a simple, painless and effective check used by midwives and doctors to assess a newborn's health.

areola the ring of pigmented skin surrounding a nipple.

artificial rupture of membranes (ARM) often known as 'breaking the waters', this is a stage of induction when the midwife makes a small nick in the amniotic sac that is holding the baby.

assisted delivery delivery of the baby with the use of forceps or ventouse.

baby blues a type of depression some women experience after having a baby. It can develop within the first six weeks of giving birth, but is often not apparent until around six months.

'back to back' presentation when the baby's spine is lying against the mother's spine.

bag of waters *see* amniotic sac.

birth canal the passageway from the womb through the cervix, the vagina and the vulva through which a fetus passes during birth.

birthing centre run by midwives without the medical facilities of a hospital. It can be next to a main hospital maternity unit ('alongside') or completely separate from hospital ('freestanding').

birth plan a written record of what the mother would like to happen during her labour and after the baby is born.

Braxton Hicks contractions the occasional hardenings of the woman's stomach during pregnancy in preparation for birth. These may be mistaken for the contractions of labour.

breaking the waters also known as artificial rupture of membranes (or ARM), this is a stage of induction when the midwife makes a small nick in the amniotic sac that is holding the baby.

breastfeeding feeding a baby with milk at the mother's breast.

breech position before birth, when a baby's head is up, with their bottom in the mother's pelvis.

caesarean an operation to deliver the baby through a cut made in the mother's abdomen rather than the baby being delivered vaginally.

catheter a flexible tube inserted through a narrow opening into a body cavity, particularly the bladder, for removing fluid.

cervix the narrow neck-like passage forming the lower end of the womb.

cholasma or 'the mask of pregnancy' a skin discolouration on the mother's face during pregnancy. This should return to normal after birth.

chorionic villus sampling (CVS) a diagnostic test to detect disorders such as Down's syndrome in the fetus. It is done by taking a sample of tissue from the chorionic villi (growths in the placenta). The test is only likely to be done if a screening test indicated there may be a problem or if the baby is deemed at high risk of an abnormality. The test is usually done before 14 weeks of pregnancy.

chromosomal abnormality occurs when there is an error in cell division, which results in a baby being born with a genetic condition, an example of which is Down's syndrome.

colostrum the first breast milk, a sweet thick substance that precedes breast milk and gives the newborn baby a host of nutrients and antibodies.

contraception (postnatal) mini-pill (progesterone-only) for use while breastfeeding; progesterone-only implants or injection; copper coil (IUD); hormone coil (IUS); barrier methods (condoms/femidoms).

contraction the muscles of the womb tightening and relaxing during labour, pushing the baby down and opening the cervix.

cord *see* umbilical cord.

crowning when the baby's head has passed through the birth canal and the top or 'crown' is visible at the vaginal opening.

crown-to-rump length measurement of the baby from the top of its head to the buttocks.

diamorphine an opiate that can be given in labour to help women cope with the pain.

diastasis recti a condition when the abdominal muscles have separated during pregnancy.

dilation as labour starts, the cervix begins to soften and slowly open, eventually to about 10 cm which is big enough to deliver the baby.

Doppler machine a machine that uses ultrasonic sound waves to listen to the baby's heartbeat.

doula a woman who provides general help for new mothers.

Down's syndrome a genetic condition that causes some level of learning disability and characteristic physical features.

early labour the early stage of labour when contractions begin and the cervix starts to soften and dilate to 3-4 cm.

eclampsia a life-threatening condition in pregnancy which can cause seizures or coma.

ectopic pregnancy this is when the embryo implants outside the uterus. This pregnancy is not viable and urgent treatment is needed for the safety of the mother.

ECV (external cephalic version) the procedure of attempting to turn the baby in the womb so the baby is in a better position for delivery.

embryo a term describing a baby in the womb from conception up to nine weeks of development.

en caul birth (or mermaid birth) when a baby is born in its amniotic sac.

endometrium the mucous membrane lining the womb.

engaged when the baby's head drops down into the mother's pelvis.

engorgement when the breasts become swollen and uncomfortable, relieved by breastfeeding the baby.

epidural a procedure to take away the pain of labour by injecting local anaesthetic into the spinal fluid.

episiotomy a small cut made to the opening of the vagina to assist delivery and avoid tearing during birth.

failure to progress if labour isn't moving forwards according to the guidelines, an assisted delivery (forceps or ventouse), or a caesarean section, may be advised.

fetal distress the presence of signs in a pregnant woman – before or during childbirth – that suggest that the fetus may not be well. These may be: moving around less than usual; meconium (fetus's poo) showing in the waters when they break.

fetal heart rate regularly checked using Doppler ultrasound machines throughout the pregnancy, and continuously at the birth if medical intervention is needed.

fetus a term describing a baby in the womb from 9 weeks up to 24 weeks of development.

first stage of labour another name for the active stage of birth, when the cervix dilates from 4–10 cm and contractions come regularly at 3–5-minute intervals.

folic acid studies have shown that if taken while trying to conceive, and continued for the first 12 weeks of pregnancy when the baby's spine is developing, this dramatically reduces the risk of spinal cord abnormalities.

fontanelles soft spots on the top and back of the baby's head, where the skull bones have not yet met.

forceps smooth metal instruments that look like large tongs used to assist delivery by locking on to the baby's head.

full-term 37 weeks is considered 'term', which means if a baby was born now it would not be premature.

gas and air otherwise known as nitrous oxide or laughing gas, this gas is inhaled as a form of pain relief during labour.

general practitioner (GP) a doctor based in the community who treats patients with minor or chronic illnesses and refers those with serious conditions to a hospital.

haemorrhagic disease of the newborn an early bleeding problem that can occur in newborns but can be entirely prevented by giving the baby vitamin K.

haemorrhoids painful or itchy swollen veins protruding from the anus that can occur in pregnancy but should disappear a few weeks after the baby is born.

HCG short for 'human chorionic gonadotrophin', this is a hormone produced during pregnancy.

home birth has the advantage of the mother feeling more relaxed, which may lead to an easier birth, but the disadvantage of being at a distance from hospital facilities should urgent medical attention be needed.

hyperemesis gravidarum an extreme form of morning sickness when you are vomiting so much that you can't keep much inside.

hypnobirthing a technique of using self-hypnosis to remain relaxed during labour. This is said to naturally reduce the adrenaline in the body so that the labour hormones oxytocin, prostaglandin and endorphins can relax the muscles, easing labour.

incontinence leakage of urine after giving birth, can be avoided or alleviated by doing regular pelvic floor exercises.

induction the artificial starting of labour by: membrane sweep; insertion of a prostaglandin tablet, pessary or gel into the vagina; artificial rupture of membranes (ARM); administering Syntocinon through an intravenous drip.

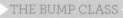

jaundice a condition that makes the skin and the whites of the eyes go yellow, caused by having too much of the pigment bilirubin.

labour the period that immediately precedes a baby's birth, in which the waters break and contractions start, these gradually increasing in intensity and frequency. *Also see* stages of labour.

lanugo the fine hair that covers the body of the fetus.

latching on the baby being properly positioned for his breastfeed, ensuring his mouth takes in the areola and that the nipple is near the roof of his mouth.

latent phase another name for early labour, when the cervix is starting to soften and dilates to 3–4 cm.

linea alba the (invisible) line that runs down the midline of the body between the belly button and pubic bone.

linea negra a dark line that runs down the midline of the body during pregnancy. This is actually the darkening of the linea alba and it should return to normal after birth.

lochia the normal discharge from the uterus after childbirth.

mastitis an infection of the breast tissue usually triggered by a blocked milk duct.

meconium the dark green sticky substance that is passed as the baby's first poo. It is made up of secretions from the baby's bowel, gall bladder and liver, as well as dead skin cells and the remains of the lanugo.

membranes the amniotic sac that surrounds an unborn baby.

mermaid birth (or en caul birth) when a baby is born in its amniotic sac.

midwife a person, usually – but not always – a woman, who is trained to assist women in childbirth.

miscarriage the loss of a pregnancy during the first 23 weeks.

morning sickness feelings of nausea, with or without vomiting, that often accompanies early pregnancy. It is usually at its worst between weeks 4 and 12.

Moro reflex a natural reflex that makes babies' arms fly out to the sides, usually in response to a sudden noise.

moxibustion performed by an acupuncturist without the use of needles, with the aim of getting a breech baby to turn spontaneously.

mucus plug fills and seals the cervical canal during pregnancy and acts as a protective barrier by deterring the passage of bacteria into the uterus.

nausea a feeling of sickness which often precedes vomiting.

nuchal scan the first scan at around 12 weeks that combines ultrasound scanning and a blood test to determine the risk of the fetus having any abnormalities and checks the fetus is growing well.

obstetrics the branch of medicine and surgery concerned with childbirth and midwifery.

paediatrician a medical practitioner specialising in children and their diseases.

pelvic floor muscles run from the pubic bone to the base of the spine. They are shaped like a sling and hold the pelvic organs (uterus, vagina, bowel and bladder) in place. They relax at the same time as the bladder contracts (tightens) to let urine out.

pelvis a basin-shaped structure of the skeleton, composed in humans of the hipbones on the sides, the pubis in front, and the sacrum and coccyx behind, that rests on the lower limbs and supports the spinal column.

perineal massage can reduce the chances of tearing during the baby's birth or the need for episiotomy if carried out for three to five weeks before delivery.

perineum the tissue between the back wall of the vagina and the rectum (back passage).

pethidine an opiate that can be given in labour to help women cope with the pain.

placenta an organ attached to the lining of the womb during pregnancy, nourishing and maintaining the fetus through the umbilical cord.

placenta praevia when the placenta sits low in the womb and is partially or totally covering the cervix.

postnatal relating to the time after birth.

postnatal depression mood changes, irritability and episodes of tearfulness, more persistent than the 'baby blues'.

postnatal period begins immediately after the birth of a child and extends to about six weeks.

pre-eclampsia a dangerous condition in pregnancy characterised by high blood pressure and protein in the urine.

pregnancy test markers that indicate pregnancy are found in urine and blood, and pregnancy tests require sampling one of these substances.

premature baby an infant born earlier than usual, before 37 weeks.

PROM (premature rupture of membranes) when waters break early, before 37 weeks.

rectum the final section of the large intestine, terminating at the anus.

relaxin from about week 8 of pregnancy, a hormone called relaxin is released which makes muscles, joints and ligaments more supple, allowing the mother's body to accommodate her growing baby.

rupture of membranes the waters breaking, indicating that labour is about to begin.

second stage of labour the stage when the mother pushes and delivers the baby.

show (bloody) when the plug of mucus from the mother's cervix comes away, up to ten days before labour starts. This is a clear jelly-like substance that is often tinged with streaks of blood.

stages of labour (1) early labour or the 'latent stage'; (2) active labour; (3) pushing; (4) delivery of the placenta.

stretch marks narrow streaks or lines that occur on the surface of the skin, the result of the skin suddenly stretching as in pregnancy. Often red or purple to start with, before gradually fading to a silvery-white colour.

sweeping of the membranes when the midwife attempts to trigger labour by stretching the cervix and separating it from the membranes containing the baby.

TENS machine a machine that emits small electrical pulses to help reduce the pain of labour.

term from 37 weeks the mother is considered 'term' and the baby, if born now, is no longer premature.

third stage of labour the stage of labour when the mother delivers the placenta.

transitional labour the stage when women who have been labouring really well suddenly think they can no longer cope. Physiologically, it's when a woman is transitioning into the pushing stage.

trimester pregnancy is dated over 40 weeks and consists of three trimesters – three lots of roughly three months.

ultrasound scans use sound waves to build a picture of the baby in the womb, which can be viewed on a screen.

umbilical cord connects an unborn baby to its mother. Oxygen and nutrients from the mother's bloodstream pass through the placenta into the cord and into the baby's bloodstream. The average cord is about 50 cm (20 inches) long.

uterus the organ in the lower body of a woman where offspring are conceived and in which they develop before birth.

vagina a tube about 8 cm long, which leads from the cervix (the neck of the womb) down to the vulva.

vaginal birth the birth of a baby through the vagina.

varicose veins swollen and enlarged veins, usually blue or dark purple, that can appear on the legs during pregnancy.

VBAC (vaginal birth after caesarean) having a baby vaginally when the mother has previously had at least one baby by caesarean section. Labour is considered to be higher risk, so will be checked more closely and more often, with continuous electronic fetal monitoring.

ventouse a small round cup that uses suction to assist the delivery of the baby.

vernix a thick white greasy substance that protects the baby in the womb.

vulva a woman's external sexual organs, these being the opening of the vagina, the inner and outer lips (labia) and the clitoris.

water birth a birth in which the mother spends the final stages of labour in a birthing pool, with delivery taking place either in or out of the water.

womb *see* uterus.

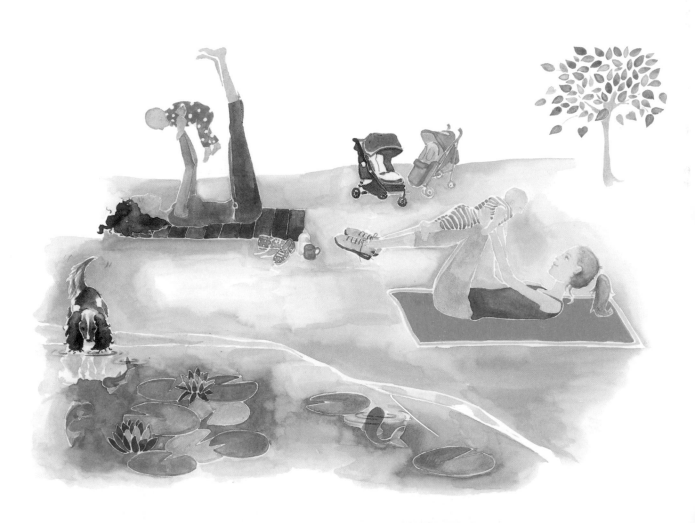

Index

THE BUMP CLASS

THE BUMP CLASS

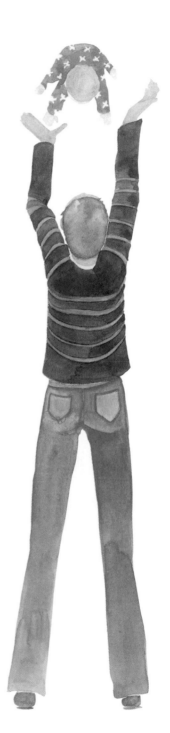

INDEX

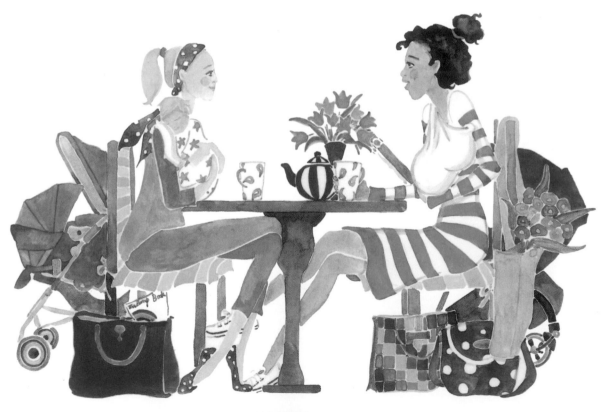

THE BUMP CLASS

Acknowledgements

This book has been a labour of love, but is by no means a work attributable entirely to its authors. They say that behind every successful man is a strong woman; in our case we couldn't have done this without the expert team behind us.

Thank you to the professionals who gave this book the gravitas that was so important to us from the outset.

To Lorin Lakasing, consultant obstetrician, for taking precious time in between looking after high risk pregnancies and her own family, to read and advise us on various chapters on medical intervention.

To Yiannis Ioannou, consultant paediatrician, for advising us and commenting on various issues in the postnatal section with unparalleled expertise, wit and humour.

To Camilla Lawrence, our Women's Health Physiotherapist, a key member of our team from the beginning, for your sanguine advice. Our pelvic floors have never been stronger!

To Liz Noonan and Elidh Parslow, our trusted midwives. Not only did you play a crucial role in each of our pregnancies and births, but your practical advice peppered with fascinating anecdotes drawn from years of experience makes our birth chapters (and Bump Classes) invaluable and great fun.

To Geraldine Miskin whose gentle yet honest and skilled approach to breastfeeding has helped Bump Class girls in their hundreds and whose book is a great complement to this one.

To our agents Charlotte Robertson and Rosemary Scoular at United Agents, for believing in us and The Bump Class and giving us confidence that the literary world would be interested in our book.

To the team at Ebury, in particular Lizzy Gray and Louise McKeever, for your patience, encouragement and attention to detail. We hope you think it was worth the wait!

To our nannies Chloe and Paulya, the essential ingredient for every working mother. Thank you for being so loving to, and so loved by, our children. Knowing our children are happy, safe and adored by you has made it possible for us to create this. We are forever grateful.

To all the girls we have met through The Bump Class, thank you for trusting us to teach you what we felt you needed to know, for your honesty, wit and enthusiasm that make every class different as well as great fun and for sharing your experiences with us. It is such a privilege for us to be a part of your pregnancies and births. One of you wrote this to us and it still brings tears to our eyes. 'You were both real inspirations to me during the course … in a way all of these babies belong to you.'

To our parents for encouraging us to start The Bump Class and for being quite the best grandparents possible. Mummy, you told us in the early days of sleep deprived fog that being a mother was the best thing we'd ever do … we weren't convinced at the time, but (as usual) you were right.

To our sister Olivia, for entertaining our unruly rabble, bringing your energy and sense of humour to days when we were so tired we could hardly walk. Also for your literary expertise, contacts and wry advice when it came to thinking about a book. We look forward to having you in the class …

To our husbands, Rupert and Den, the sometimes rocky road of parenthood would not be half as fun without you both. Thank you for being such wonderful husbands and enthusiastic, fun and energetic fathers. Seeing the sheer joy you both derive from the children is an inspiration to us.

About The Bump Class

The Bump Class was conceived one wet New Year's day by sisters Dr Chiara Hunt and Marina Fogle. Having seen the effect of ill preparation, myths, stigma and fear on pregnant women and young mothers, Chiara and Marina were certain that an honest antenatal class, led by engaging and experienced professionals, would be a runaway sensation. The first course started in early 2013 and became an instant success. The reputation of The Bump Class continues to grow and each year hundreds of women are grateful for what they feel is the best preparation possible for the birth of their children. www.thebumpclass.com

Marina Fogle is married to the adventurer Ben Fogle. They have two children, Ludo and Iona, and in spite of tragedy (her son Willem was stillborn in 2014), Marina has become motherhood's biggest advocate. As well as teaching at The Bump Class, she juggles writing for *The Telegraph* about pregnancy and motherhood with looking after her children and two dogs. Marina and her family live in West London.

Dr Chiara Hunt, MBBS BSc MRCGP DFSRH, studied at Imperial College and then worked at St Mary's Paddington and the Chelsea and Westminster in London, before quickly realising that her special interest lay in in treating families. After becoming a mother to Otto and Ivy, Chiara became even more determined to develop an expertise in treating pregnant and postnatal women and their babies. Her working life is divided between seeing patients at her London practice and teaching at The Bump Class. She lives in London with her two children and her husband.

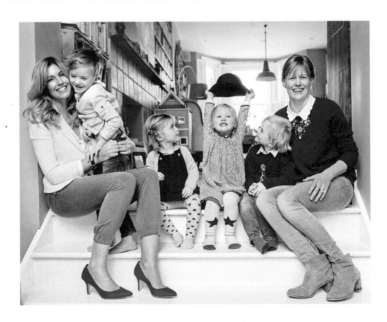